WINSTON

# STUDY GUIDE
## TO ACCOMPANY
# HEALTH INFORMATION:
## *Management of a Strategic Resource*
### *Second Edition*

**ELLEN JACOBS**, MEd, RHIA
**MARY ALICE HANKEN**, PhD, RHIA
**BEVERLI H. REDING**, PhD, RHIA

**Managing Editor**
**Mervat Abdelhak, PhD, RHIA**
Department Chair and Associate Professor
Health Information Management
School of Health and Rehabilitation Sciences
University of Pittsburgh
Pittsburgh, PA

**Editors**
**Sara Grostick, MA, RHIA**
Director, Health Information Management Program
and Associate Professor
School of Health Related Professions
University of Alabama at Birmingham
Birmingham, AL

**Mary Alice Hanken, PhD, RHIA**
Independent Consultant; Senior Lecturer
Health Information Administration Program
School of Public Health and Community Medicine
University of Washington
Seattle, WA

**Ellen Jacobs, MEd, RHIA**
Director, Health Information Management
Program and Associate Professor
College of Saint Mary
Omaha, NE

**W.B. SAUNDERS COMPANY**
A Harcourt Health Sciences Company
Philadelphia   London   New York   St. Louis   Sydney   Toronto

W.B. SAUNDERS COMPANY
*A Harcourt Health Sciences Company*

The Curtis Center
Independence Square West
Philadelphia, Pennsylvania 19106-3399

Study Guide to Accompany
Health Information: Management of a Strategic Resource, Second Edition  ISBN 0-7216-8675-3

Copyright © 2001, 1996 by W.B. Saunders Company

All rights reserved. No part of this publication may be reproduced or transmitted in any form or by any means, electronic or mechanical, including photocopy, recording, or any information storage and retrieval system, without permission in writing from the publisher, except that, until further notice, instructors requiring their students to purchase HEALTH INFORMATION: MANAGEMENT OF A STRATEGIC RESOURCE, Second Edition by Mervat Abdelhak, Sara Grostick, Mary Alice Hankin and Ellen B. Jacobs, may reproduce the contents or parts thereof for instructional purposes, provided each copy contains a proper copyright notice as follows: © 2001 by W.B. Saunders Company.

Printed in the United States of America.

Last digit is the print number: 9 8 7 6 5 4 3 2 1

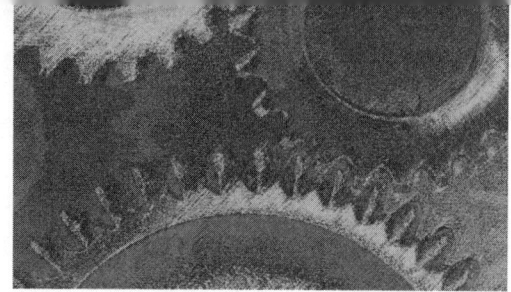

# TABLE OF CONTENTS

Introduction ..................................................................................................... 1

## Section One: Study and Test-Taking Techniques

**Study Techniques** ........................................................................................... 5

**Test-Taking Principles** ..................................................................................... 6

**Purpose of Review Questions** ...................................................................... 12

**Preparing for Chapter Reviews** .................................................................... 12

**Pretest Reviews** ............................................................................................ 13

**Chapter Reviews** ......................................................................................... 13

**Preparing Performance Grids** ...................................................................... 13

**Working with Critical Competence Questions** ............................................. 14

**AHIMA Domains and Subdomains** ............................................................. 15

    Guide to Domains and Subdomains for the Registered Health
    Information Technician ............................................................................ 16

    Guide to Domains and Subdomains for the Registered Health
    Information Administration ...................................................................... 21

## Section Two: Review Questions and Assignments by Chapter

**Foundations of Health Information Management**
    Chapter 1: Health Care Systems ............................................................. 27
    Chapter 2: The Health Information Management Profession ................. 39

## Health Care Data

- Chapter 3: Data Collection Standards ............................................. 51
- Chapter 4: Data Quality and Technology ....................................... 71
- Chapter 5: Data Access and Retention .......................................... 89
- Chapter 6: Coding, Classification, and Reimbursement Systems ................. 107

## Data Management and Use

- Chapter 7: Registries ............................................................ 121
- Chapter 8: Statistics ............................................................ 131
- Chapter 9: Research and Epidemiology ......................................... 147
- Chapter 10: Quality Management and Clinical Outcomes ....................... 159
- Chapter 11: Health Law Concepts and Practices ................................ 177

## Management

- Chapter 12: Principles of Management .......................................... 191
- Chapter 13: Operational Management ........................................... 203
- Chapter 14: Human Resource Management ..................................... 227
- Chapter 15: Financial Management .............................................. 257

## Information Systems

- Chapter 16: Technology, Applications, and Security ............................ 271
- Chapter 17: Electronic Health Records: A Unifying Principle ................... 279
- Chapter 18: Information Systems Life Cycle .................................... 287

# Section Three: How to Prepare for Certification

- Introduction and Application ..................................................... 301
- Certification Examination Content ............................................... 302
- Certification Examination Cost .................................................. 303
- Certification Examination Scoring ............................................... 303
- Preparing for Certification—Before the Exam ................................... 303
- Preparing for Certification—During the Exam ................................... 305

# Section Four: How to Interpret Your Examination Readiness

- Using Performance Grids ........................................................ 309

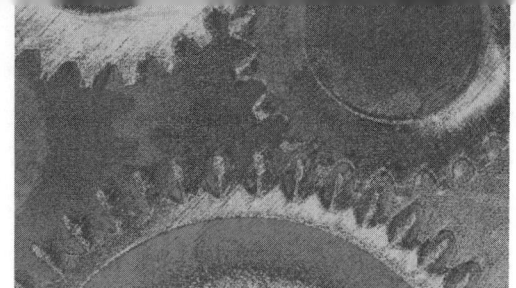

# CD-ROM TABLE OF CONTENTS
## *SELECT ASSIGNMENTS*

### Chapter 1: Health Care Systems
- 1-4: Internet Resources
- 1-6: Health Care Organizations/Agencies
- 1-8: Insurance Grid
- 1-9: Medicare

### Chapter 2: The Health Information Management Profession
- 2-1: AHIMA Web Site
- 2-2: JCAHO Resources

### Chapter 3: Data Collection Standards
- 3-5: Uniform Hospital Discharge Data Set (UHDDS)
- 3-9: Evaluation of Content of an Inpatient Acute Care Hospital Record
- 3-10: Ongoing Record Review
- 3-11: Delinquent Record Statistics
- 3-14: Thought Questions

### Chapter 4: Data Quality and Technology
- 4-3: Computer Topic Presentation
- 4-7: Incident Report Data Entry Form
- 4-8: Event and Validation Checks
- 4-10: Forms Design
- 4-11: Annual Report—Word Processing

### Chapter 5: Data Access and Retention
- 5-5: Hill-Burton Community Hospital—Pharmacy
- 5-6: Modern Clinic—Transcription
- 5-7: Modern Clinic—Record Tracking System
- 5-8: Advanced Technology Hospital (ATH) On-Line Optical Image Based Patient Record—Costs
- 5-9: Advanced Technology Hospital (ATH) On-Line Optical Image Based Patient Record—Personnel

5-15: Quad State Medical Center—Record Retention
5-16: Pediatricians' Office—A New Alphabetical File
5-18: Thought Questions

## Chapter 6: Coding, Classification, and Reimbursement Systems
6-1: Classification Exercise
6-4: Professional Practice Experience: Assessing the Quality of Coded Data
6-5: Consulting
6-6: Hiring a Coder

## Chapter 7: Registries
7-2: Cancer Registry Accession List
7-3: Primary Site Table

## Chapter 8: Statistics
8-3: Length of Stay Statistics
8-4: Thought Questions

## Chapter 9: Research and Epidemiology
9-1: Thought Questions
9-5: HIM Use of Descriptive Research
9-10: Data Collection
9-11: Data Analysis
9-12: Prospective Study on Data Trends

## Chapter 10: Quality Management and Clinical Outcomes
10-1: Internet Scavenger Hunt
10-2: Peer Review Organization Information on the Web
10-3: Data Collection on Patient Falls
10-6: Using Run Charts to Tackle the Record Delinquency Problem

## Chapter 11: Health Law Concepts and Practices
11-1: Reference Guide
11-3: Development of a Release of Information Database
11-4: Release of Information Scenarios
11-8: Thought Questions

## Chapter 12: Principles of Management
12-4: Medical Associates, Inc.
12-5: South Land Managed Care
12-6: Medical Laboratory Enterprises
12-7: Valley Behavioral Health Hospital

## Chapter 13: Operational Management

- 13-4: Professional Practice: Systems Flowcharts
- 13-5: Professional Practice: Operations/Procedure Flowchart
- 13-6: Professional Practice: Movement Diagram
- 13-7: Group Exercise: Decision Matrix
- 13-8: Group Exercise: Project Management
- 13-10: PERT Network

## Chapter 14: Human Resource Management

- 14-3: Accommodating Gender Preferences: Sports or Soaps?
- 14-4: Entrepreneurs With Medical Language Specialists
- 14-7: Changes at Happy Trails Health Center
- 14-17: Guilty Until Proven Innocent?
- 14-19: Work from Home: Will it Work?

## Chapter 15: Financial Management

- 15-2: Graphic Representation of Data and Data Analysis
- 15-5: Variance Analysis
- 15-6: Case Mix Analysis
- 15-8: Personal Balance Sheet

## Chapter 16: Technology, Applications, and Security

- 16-4: HTML/XML Fact Sheet

## Chapter 17: Electronic Health Records: A Unifying Principle

- 17-2: Forecast Document
- 17-3: In-Service Program on Confidentiality of Electronic Health Records
- 17-7: Personal Strategic Plan
- 17-10: Thought Questions

## Chapter 18: Information Systems Life Cycle

- 18-1: Professional Practice: Analysis of Information Systems Life Cycle Stage
- 18-3: Professional Practice: Hierarchy Chart and Data Flow Diagram
- 18-4: Professional Practice: Data Dictionary
- 18-7: Implementation Plan

# CONTRIBUTING AUTHORS

**Elizabeth D. Bowman, MPA, RHIA**
Professor, Department of Health Information
  Management
University of Tennessee, Health Science Center
Memphis, Tennessee
*Chapter 6 Coding Classification and Reimbursement
  Systems*

**Jill Callahan Dennis, JD, RHIA**
Principal, Health Risk Advantage
Parker, Colorado
*Chapter 11 Health Law Concepts and Practices*

**W. Jack Duncan, PhD**
Professor and University Scholar, Graduate School of
  Management
University of Alabama at Birmingham
Birmingham, Alabama
*Chapter 12 Principles of Management*

**Shirley A. Eichenwald, RHIA**
Assistant Professor, Department of Health Information
  Management
The College of Saint Scholastica
Duluth, Minnesota
*Chapter 2 The Health Information Management
  Profession*

**Peter M. Ginter, PhD**
Professor and Chair, Health Care Organization and
  Policy
School of Public Health, University of Alabama at
  Birmingham
Birmingham, Alabama
*Chapter 12 Principles of Management*

**Darice M. Grzybowski, MA, RHIA**
Adjunct Assistant Professor, University of Illinois at
  Chicago
School of Biomedical and Health Information
  Sciences
National Manager, Health Information Management
  Industry Relations, 3M HIS
Salt Lake City, Utah
*Chapter 5 Data Access and Retention*

**Mary Alice Hanken, PhD, RHIA**
Independent Consultant; Senior Lecturer
Health Information Administration
  Program
School of Public Health and Community Medicine
University of Washington
Seattle, Washington
*Chapter 15 Financial Management*

**Anita Hazelwood, MLS, RHIA**
Associate Professor, The University of Louisiana at
  Lafayette
Lafayette, Louisiana
*Chapter 13 Operational Management*

**Loretta A. Horton, MEd, RHIA,**
Coordinator, Health Information Technology
  Program
Hutchinson Community College
Hutchinson, Kansas
*Chapter 8 Statistics*

**Merida L. Johns, PhD, RHIA**
Visiting Associate Professor and Director
Master of Science in Information Systems
  Management
Department of Information Systems and Operations
  Management
School of Business, Loyola University of Chicago
Chicago, Illinois
*Chapter 18 Information Systems Life Cycle*

**Lynn Kuehn, MS, RHIA, CCS-P**
Director of Office Operations, Children's Medical
  Group
Milwaukee, Wisconsin
*Chapter 5 Data Access and Retention*

**Mary Miller, RHIA**
Instructor, Health Information Management Program
College of Saint Mary
Omaha, Nebraska
*Chapter 6 and 8 Coding, Classification and
  Reimbursement Systems; Statistics*

**Jackie Moczygemba, MBA, RHIA**
Assistant Professor, Health Information Management Program
Southwest Texas State University
San Marcos, Texas
*Chapter 10 Quality Management and Clinical Outcomes*

**Gretchen F. Murphy, MEd, RHIA**
Director and Senior Lecturer, Health Information Administration Program
School of Public Health and Community Medicine
University of Washington
Seattle, Washington
*Chapter 17 Electronic Health Records: A Unifying Principle*

**Midge Noel Ray, MSN, RN**
Associate Professor, Health Information Management Program
Department of Critical and Diagnostic Care
University of Alabama at Birmingham
Birmingham, Alabama
*Chapter 1 Health Care Systems*

**Wesley M. Rohrer, III, PhD**
Assistant Professor and Assistant to the Dean
Department of Health Information Management
School of Health and Rehabilitation Sciences
University of Pittsburgh
Pittsburgh, Pennsylvania
*Chapter 14 Human Resource Management*

**Elaine Rubinstein, PhD**
Adjunct Assistant Professor
Department of Health Information Management and Research
Specialist, Office of Measurement and Evaluation of Teaching
University of Pittsburgh
Pittsburgh, Pennsylvania
*Chapter 8 Statistics*

**Melissa Saul, MS**
Adjunct Assistant Professor, Health Information Management
School of Health and Rehabilitation Sciences
University of Pittsburgh
Director, Project Engineering
Medical Archival Systems, Inc., UPMC Health System
Pittsburgh, Pennsylvania
*Chapter 16 Technology, Applications, and Security*

**Donna J. Slovensky, PhD, RHIA**
Associate Professor and Director, BS in Allied Health Program
School of Health Related Professions
University of Alabama at Birmingham
Birmingham, Alabama
*Chapter 10 Quality Management and Clinical Outcomes*

**Mary Spivey Teslow, MLIS, RHIA**
Program Coordinator, Health Information Management
Broward Community College
Fort Lauderdale, Florida
*Chapters 3 and 4 Data Collection Standards; Data Quality and Technology*

**Carol Venable, MPH, RHIA**
Associate Professor and Department Head
The University of Louisiana at Lafayette
Lafayette, Louisiana
*Chapter 13 Operational Management*

**Sue Watkins, RHIA, CTR**
Director, Health Information Technology and Cancer Information Management Programs
Santa Barbara City College
Santa Barbara, California
*Chapter 7 Registries*

**Valerie J.M. Watzlaf, PhD, RHIA**
Associate Professor, Department of Health Information Management
School of Health and Rehabilitation Sciences
University of Pittsburgh
Pittsburgh, Pennsylvania
*Chapters 8 and 9 Statistics; Research and Epidemiology*

**Diane Weiss, RHIA**
Clinical Faculty, University of Washington, Seattle
Associate Faculty, Shoreline Community College
Shoreline, Washington
Consultant, DM Weiss & Associates
Seattle, Washington
*Chapter 15 Financial Management*

**Donna J. Wilde, MPA, RHIA**
Director and Professor, Health Care Information Programs
Shoreline Community College
Seattle, Washington
*Chapters 3 and 4 Data Collection Standards; Data Quality and Technology*

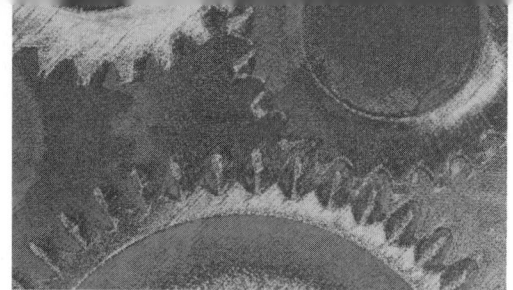

# INTRODUCTION

The *Study Guide to Accompany Health Information: Management of a Strategic Resource* is designed to involve the user in the learning process. Individual learning styles vary from those who learn best by writing, reading, listening, to those who learn by doing. Many people feel they learn and retain material longer from "doing" activities. This guide is designed to emphasize the doing and the application of the knowledge in the book *Health Information: Management of a Strategic Resource*. By using this guide, you become a "hands-on" learner engaged in using and applying critical thinking skills to the knowledge gained throughout.

This Study Guide can be used in many ways: (1) as assignments by the instructor in residential or distance learning courses that either are or are not using *Health Information* as a text; (2) as self-study to see if you are mastering the concepts of the course; (3) as part of an in-service training program in a health information practice setting.

The concepts and ideas used in the Study Guide follow the sequence of chapters and use the same titles as the book *Health Information: Management of a Strategic Resource*. For each chapter, the Study Guide contains Review Questions and Assignments.

## Review Questions

Each chapter has 10 pretest and 10 chapter review questions. The chapter review questions as well as 30 additional questions for each chapter are featured on the CD-ROM found in the back of this guide. Use these to assess your knowledge before and after reading each chapter.

## Assignments

To accommodate and capitalize on the various learning styles, this Study Guide offers a variety of ways to apply the concepts addressed in this book. These include the following:

- **Case Studies/Scenarios**
  Several chapters involve scenarios developed by the contributors from real-life situations. By simulating real-life situations, the scenarios will stimulate thought and discussion.
- **Thought Questions**
  Critical analysis and problem solving are abilities that are needed in today's and tomorrow's health information practice. Responding to these questions requires you to think, analyze, and problem solve using the concepts presented in the book.

Copyright © 2001 by W.B. Saunders Company. All rights reserved.

- **Group Exercises**
  Another valued capability in health care is to be a participatory member of a team. Group exercises give you the opportunity to work with your peers in this manner.
- **Professional Practice Experiences**
  Activities that are best completed in a live health information management situation are labeled as professional practice experiences. These activities take on different forms and outcomes depending on the place chosen to complete them.

This Study Guide is the collective thought of an imaginative group of contributors (listed on the contributors' page) and editors. It would not have been possible without them. It is our hope that this Study Guide will enhance the learning process, complement *Health Information: Management of a Strategic Resource*, and improve health information management education and practice.

The Editors

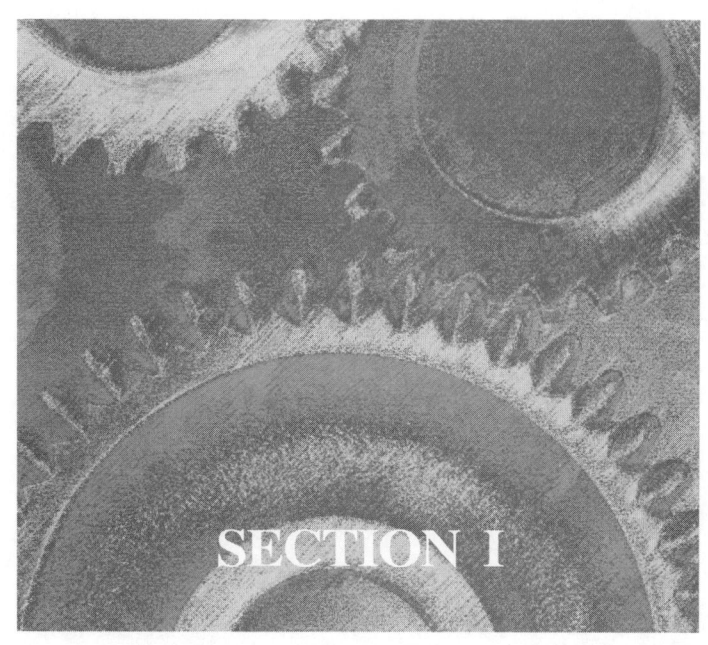

# SECTION I

# STUDY AND TEST-TAKING TECHNIQUES

# Study Techniques

(Note: While this section is primarily for students, health information practitioners may also gain considerable insight into mastery preparation by reviewing the information that is supplied.)

Before attempting to use this Study Guide, evaluate your approach to studying. Is your study plan working for you, or can it be improved? The following discussion may assist in refining your approach to studying.

1. **Scan all your learning resources for a unit.**

Survey the chapter, paying attention to headings, subheadings, topic sentences, and key concepts. Include your course assignments, handouts, notes, and this Study Guide (corresponding also to the learning unit in progress). When you get a broad view of the whole, the parts take on added meaning—how they all fit together. This helps to eliminate surprises and to give you a feeling for the breadth of the task.

2. **Study the objectives for each chapter.**

Focus on the verb. Are you expected to define, list, describe, or recognize? Whatever the verb used, it will suggest how you may be tested. Short essay questions requiring a one-sentence response may be used to define terms; matching questions to identify definitions, principles or concepts. Regular essay questions may be used for asking your description of a broader concept or principle, or your justification for a response, such as can be answered in one or more brief paragraphs. Short completion questions may be used when the objective asks you to list, name, or identify something. The types of questions to be used in this Study Guide are discussed elsewhere in this section.

Always write out answers to objectives and be sure to be guided by any additional objectives supplied by your instructor; verify with your instructor all the chapter objectives for which you are responsible. Answering objectives can be done concurrently with reading the chapter, for the process can enhance your comprehension of the material.

3. **Read the entire textbook chapter, including key terms.**

Glance over the chapter outline, chapter objectives, and key terms before proceeding in reading to determine the important subject matter requiring significant attention. The review questions emphasizes that foundational content, particularly the objectives. (Note: Reading is a most important phase of learning that requires the highest level of concentration. Any outside noise can subconsciously be distracting, thereby negatively impacting your concentration without your consciously realizing it. Attempt to find the quietest place for this exercise.)

4. **Underscore or highlight principles, theories, purposes, rationales, and basic concepts that correspond with the objectives.**

This process emphasizes their learning in the context in which they have been written in the text.

## 5. Develop mini-outlines of a principle or related principles that appear over the course of several pages in the textbook.

Use 3 x 5 cards or regular notebook paper if it would facilitate storage. For example, chapter objective 3-8 in Chapter 3, Data Collection Standards, states "Define the 10 characteristics of data quality." As you are reading the chapter, you discover that ten (10) characteristics of data quality are discussed over 2 to 3 pages. They are accuracy, accessibility, comprehensiveness, consistency, currency, definition, granularity, precision, relevancy, and timeliness. From this, your mini-outline can illustrate the fundamental information, and by alphabetizing the characteristics, facilitate easier recall of the information in its total context:

**Mini-Outline**
**Objective 3-8:**
Characteristics of data quality—meaning data has quality when it is:
1. accurate
2. accessible
3. comprehensive
4. consistent
5. current
6. defined
7. granular
8. precise
9. relevant
10. timely
    (Note: See key terms for definitions)

Since definitions are provided for these terms in the Glossary of the text, a note to yourself on this point is added to the mini-outline.

## 6. Organize all of your learning materials.

Get them all together for each chapter: answers to objectives, lecture notes, lab exercises, and handouts. (Note: Some students assemble all materials from all sources in a three-ring notebook for each subject unit. Upon preparing for finals and the certification examination, they simply review the same material in the order they learned it originally without any additional organization required).

## 7. Begin your review early.

Review is designed to assist in recall; it cannot he accomplished hastily. Even if you recall information easily, review in order to "over-learn." It builds confidence, reduces anxiety, and should translate into correct application.

# Test-Taking Principles

In addition to subject preparation, taking and passing examinations is dependent upon other factors. The following principles are general and not necessarily unique and applicable only to this Study Guide or subject matter. These principles are suggested to act as guidelines, and not absolutes, in choosing the best response for a question.

## 1. Find out how the test is scored.

This may be stated in the test directions, in the course syllabus, or in preprinted test materials. Determine if the exam score is based on the total number of questions on the test or the number of questions answered. This will tell you whether guessing of failing to answer all the questions will hurt your score. Knowing the scoring methodology enables you to set your test-writing strategy in advance.

## 2. Find out the type of questions to be asked.

Again, this is important in developing your studying strategy. If the test is all essay, your study approach may be different than if it were all multiple choice.

## 3. Become familiar with the types of questions.

In this Study Guide, six types of questions are used.

### Multiple Choice Questions

A question is asked in a stem followed by one correct or best answer and three distracters or wrong answers. Oftentimes, a distracter may be partially correct, in which case, it is not the best answer. Be sure to compare all four or five alternative choices against the stem of the question—not to each other—before making your choice.

Examples:

Of the following employees, which provides the required information as an intermediary between someone needing data (customer) and the data sources (supplier)?
a. data entry operator
b. data broker
c. data query engineer
d. data technician

Answer: b

Which of the following is a research study design that deals only with survivors; is not effective in studying rare diseases; and will often miss an epidemic?
a. case-control study
b. prospective study
c. cross-sectional study
d. clinical trial

Answer: c

### True/False Questions

This type of question asks if a statement is true. The entire statement must be true to denote true, otherwise, it is not true, but is false. Determine the correct answer only by the information stated; do not attempt to read into the question information that is not there.

Examples:

The current title of the national organization of Registered Health Information Technicians (RHITs) and Registered Health Information Administrators (RHIAs) is the American Medical Record Association.
a. True
b. False

Answer: b

An executive information system is a type of decision support system.

a. True
b. False

Answer: b

## Yes/No Question

This type of question asks your agreement or opinion about information. If your agreement is yes, select yes; if your agreement is no, select no.

Examples:

A student in a health care professional training program enters the HIM department and asks for Mr. Rocky State's most recent health record. Since the student is on clinical experience, she should be permitted access to Mr. State's patient record. Do you agree?

a. Yes
b. No

Answer: b

The human resources director is urging the HIM department director to develop a transcriptionist training program. She has argued that there is no capital investment involved in the development of the new service because the dictation and transcription equipment is already in place. Do you agree that this is an accurate statement?

a. Yes
b. No

Answer: b

## Problem Solving Questions

A question provides a scenario or brief description of an incident, situation, or problem followed by one or more questions. To answer questions correctly you need to analyze multiple facts in the scenario and draw on multiple understandings of related information in your mind in order to form a correct or best response. Sometimes, extraneous information is included in the description that is not needed for solving the problem; delete unrelated information by marking through it.

Examples:

Cafe Latte Medical Center has an average of 988 discharges per month and 341 operations. They have 183 delinquent records. Seventeen are missing history and physicals. The Medical Center received two Type I recommendations from the Joint Commission on Accreditation of Healthcare Organizations because of these deficiencies.

a. True
b. False

Answer: b

One year ago a skilled nursing facility purchased a computer system to process billing claims. Then, six months ago, the administrative office acquired a computer system to support clerical functions. Two months ago a system was purchased to assist with dietary planning.

Based on this information, which stage of Nolan's Information Life Cycle is illustrated by this organization?
a. initiation
b. expansion
c. control
d. integration
Answer:     b

## Short Answer Questions

This type of question requires a one-or-more word answer and not a complete statement, such as a sentence or brief paragraph. It is used to measure the recall of simple facts, terms, abbreviations, or symbols. Oftentimes, a term is asked for to complete a statement or sentence. You may also be asked to name or interpret diagrams, charts, or tables from given illustrations using this question type.

Examples:

1. In the health facility's patient database, there is a column for date of discharge. Give one of many edits that can be built into the computer system to help the data entry operator input that data item correctly.

    Answer: must be in MM//DD/YYYY format; may not be blank (other possibilities not mentioned here)

2. A _____ chart is a scheduling device that is a system of diagramming steps or component parts of a complex project.

    Answer:     PERT

3. Referring to the following figure, what statistical measure can best be illustrated using this type of diagram?

    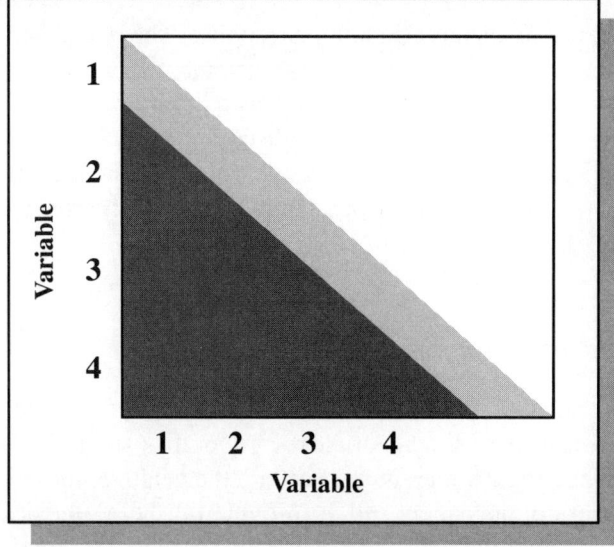

    Answer:     Correlation coefficient

## Matching Questions

This question asks the respondent to associate terms or brief statements in one column with correct descriptors of those statements in another column. In this question type, the answer is provided. Work within one column at a time, more easily the left-hand column, matching each term to the best statement in the column on the right. Place a thin pencil line through items on the right that are matched so that they will not interfere with subsequent matching. Match each item carefully, because if you change one, it may mean changing three or more. After you have marked all of the responses you are certain about, complete the matching by guessing on remaining items. (Note: Oftentimes, additional items will be provided in one or both columns for which a correct or best answer is not provided.)

Example:

Match the items in the left column with the correct descriptor in the right column. Some descriptors may not have answers.

| | | |
|---|---|---|
| _____ 1. database | a. | alpha or numeric |
| _____ 2. data file | b. | smallest unit of data |
| _____ 3. data dictionary | c. | describe objects related to a data element |
| _____ 4. data label | d. | information about stored data |
| _____ 5. data steward | e. | protects databases |
| _____ 6. data type | f. | stores data |
| | g. | data name |
| | h. | data table |

Answers:　　　1. f　　2. h　　3. d　　4. g　　5. e　　6. a

## Essay Questions

(Note: While few essay questions are utilized in this Study Guide, they are a type of question which is frequently used in test measurement to assess learning at more complex levels. For this reason, a reference is made to this type of question in the event a user of this Study Guide may be faced with organizing a response to an essay question).

This type of question requires a one-or-more paragraph response. The intent is to measure one's ability to form an accurate, yet cohesive, logical and concise statement that another person could understand—much like speaking to another person. It is suggested that on the back of the test copy you pencil a brief outline of the key points you intend to discuss; order the points by number and then formulate your response from the outline. This prevents you from accidentally dropping from the answer process a key point while discussing another point. Write clearly, concisely, and directly to the question only.

Example:

Discuss the purpose of health records.

Answer: There are several purposes the health record serves; these mentioned are but a few. The principal purpose is to provide a historical record for the patient that will serve as a foundation for continued quality care in the future. Second, the health record is maintained as a legal document for the benefit of the patient and the provider(s). Third, the health record serves as a basis for evaluating and improving the quality of care, for planning, for research, and for remuneration of patient services.

### 4. Bring to every test at least two pencils and a calculator.

Paper and notes are not generally allowed, so any calculations will have to be noted on the back of your answer sheet or in the test booklet. It is recommended that you provide yourself with an audit trail by making notes of all your math in the event you make an incorrect choice. (Note: Calculators and table surfaces may be examined by a circulating test proctor, periodically.)

### 5. Read the directions for the test carefully, and listen intently to any oral instructions given.

Generally, once an examination begins, there will be no questions answered. If you do not understand something in the directions, be sure to speak up and ask right away.

### 6. Study the answer sheet carefully and keep checking it throughout the test to make certain you are filling in the answer sheet for the question you intend to answer.

Sometimes a question number is skipped because the student intended to come back to it. Be sure to flag those questions in some way on the answer sheet so as not to inadvertently record the answer to the next successive question in its spot. Generally, answer sheets are graded by machine. Care should be given to shade in your answer completely as noted below and to erase completely, as shown:

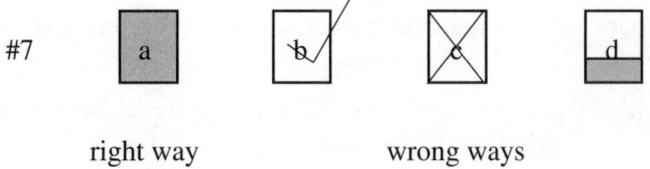

right way        wrong ways

### 7. Pace yourself by wearing a watch or sitting in view of a clock.

To prepare for this, flip through all the pages of the test before beginning to obtain an overview of its scope and layout. Familiarizing yourself with what is ahead, rather than waiting to be surprised when it may be too late, will enable you to plan your time for certain sections of the examination rather than react to a lack of sufficient time.

Many tests are not timed, but if they are, remember that the scoring may be calculated on the percent of questions you answered correctly out of the total you attempted. This means that questions you did not have time to get to will not affect your score.

### 8. Be clear about what each question is asking before attempting a response.

Reread each question and underscore key words to ensure clarity. (Note: Did you miss any of the examples above because you misread the question?)

### 9. Read each possible answer before marking your choice.

Many questions may contain two or more very similar answers from which you must choose the best or most correct answer. If you have trouble in selecting a correct or best answer, skip the question. Perhaps information within subsequent questions will trigger a correct response in your mind or provide contributing information for selecting a correct answer; be certain to mark the question you are skipping on your answer sheet as a reminder to return to it.

### 10. Before finishing an examination section, or the complete exam, go over it thoroughly to be certain all answers have been recorded.

## Purpose of Review Questions

The principal purpose of pretest and review questions is the self-examination of your mastery of the subject matter. Since answers are provided for each question in answer keys, you can determine subject areas of weakness and return to the textbook for further study. Key terms and principles are noted in bold type throughout the chapters in the textbook, enabling rapid location and reference for this purpose.

The intent of providing these review questions is not to encourage memorizing questions and answers, thinking that they may be repeated on an actual examination, but rather to help you assess and reinforce your understanding of theories, principles, concepts, and terms, including related information, so that you can be successful in answering any question on that subject correctly. This ability comes with careful reading and rereading of the textbook and collateral references, and not in becoming question dependent.

In addition to the principal purpose, additional purposes can be realized. This comprehensive review approach can also enhance performance of certain tasks and solving of simulated problems. Other purposes include:

 Increasing testing confidence
 Measuring unit examination readiness by chapter
 Enabling testing experience
 Providing an opportunity for last-minute review
 Supplying repeated review opportunities
 Increasing practice skills in certain tasks and subtasks
 Expanding knowledge and/or competence base

## Preparing for Chapter Reviews

Review questions are provided for Chapters 1–18 of the textbook. For each chapter there are a total of 50 questions, 10 of which have been organized into a Pretest Review. Subsequent to each Pretest Review is a review for each chapter composed of 10 additional questions called a Chapter Review. The CD-ROM provides a more comprehensive review for each chapter, with 30 additional questions plus a repeat of the 10 Chapter Review questions for those who prefer an electronic form of studying.

This Study Guide presupposes that you have already learned these subjects:
- Anatomy and Physiology
- Medical Terminology
- Medical Science
- Coding Practice Skills

Even though there are a wide range of topics covered in this Study Guide, topics not discussed in the textbook are also not included as review questions. Some questions test your knowledge or recall of fundamental information and principles, while others require you to apply information, principles, standards, or theory to a problem situation. Consequently, the level of difficulty increases as the content of the question moves from a recall-type question to an application or problem-solving type. The time required to answer application and problem-solving questions also increases from that required for recall-type questions. This should be taken into consideration when scheduling your time on actual examinations; the time to complete certain review questions in this Study Guide can serve as a benchmark for this purpose.

# Pretest Reviews

Each Pretest Review enables a quick self-assessment of factual knowledge pertaining to the chapter. This is accomplished by the use of true/false-type questions predominately. Use the Pretest Review after the initial reading of the chapter, preferably before pursuing any application exercises of the material. At the end of each chapter in this Study Guide is a Pretest Review Answer Key for correcting your answers. Although brief, the Pretest Review will help to alert you to any misunderstandings or principles not yet fully comprehended before you attempt the more comprehensive Chapter Review.

# Chapter Reviews

In addition to each Pretest Review are 10 Chapter Review questions utilizing the six types of questions discussed previously. Its purpose is to measure your pre-examination mastery of the chapter subject matter. The intent is to complete the Chapter Review during the process of overall examination preparation and to correct your responses promptly using the Chapter Review Answer Key located at the back of each chapter.

The results of your performance may necessitate further study of selected portions of the textbook and of lecture notes. To assist you in interpreting your performance, a Performance Grid is provided.

# Preparing Performance Grids

In Section Four of the Study Guide is a Performance Grid for you to chart your overall test performance and mastery of the textbook subject material chapter-by-chapter. The Initial Performance Grid is needed for the first-time completion of this Study Guide. The Repeat Performance Grids may be used for subsequent reviews at your own discretion, particularly if you are a student preparing for final examinations and your certification examination.

For example, assume you have just completed a Pretest Review for Chapter 1 in the textbook. You missed two questions. You record the remaining 8 which are correct in Column 2. To calculate the percent of correct responses for this Pretest Review, simply divide the number 8 by the total correct responses possible, which was 10, and record the percent in Column 3. You demonstrated a correct understanding of 80% of the subject matter.

Since this Pretest Review sample is small, it should be used only as an indication of readiness to proceed with the Chapter Review. Be sure to study the correct answers for all answers missed in the respective chapter of the text; restudy the context of the subject matter surrounding that which pertained to the questions you missed. Since your overall performance on this Pretest Review was 80% or greater, and you have studied your areas of weakness, you decide to proceed to the Chapter Review.

Assume now that you have just completed the Chapter Review. Upon correcting your Chapter Review Test with the Answer Key at the back of the chapter, you missed 3 questions. You subtract the 3 incorrect answers from the total questions in the Chapter Review, which was 10, to obtain the total number of questions you answered correctly. Record 7 correct answers in Column 5, and proceed to calculate the percent correct as you did for the Pretest Review, above. Record 70% in Column 6 on the Initial Performance Grid.

You demonstrated 70% understanding of the content of the Chapter Review. Since this is less than 75%, which is considered passing by some standards, again you should reread those portions of the chapter where the principles are discussed for each question missed. In this instance, finding out why you missed each question by simply examining a page in the textbook may be insufficient for fully grasping the material; rereading the subject matter in the broader context surrounding that which pertained to the questions missed is the recommended solution for improving your mastery.

You may want to aim at an 80% or higher mastery performance overall. It depends on the grading standards for your coursework. In this example, the student's overall chapter mastery—the Pretest Review performance plus the Chapter Review performance—was calculated to be 75%. This was obtained by summing the number correct on the Pretest Review from Column 2 with the number correct on the Chapter Review in Column 5 and dividing that sum by the total number of questions in both review tests which is 30 (Column 1 + Column 4). This overall percent is recorded in Column 7. Aiming for a higher mastery than needed to pass a unit test or a final examination helps to establish a margin for error due to carelessness, misreading, or some other reason. Aiming at 100% mastery is not an unreasonable review goal. Consider it an opportunity. This same formula can be applied to the additional questions on the CD-ROM.

# Working With Critical Competence Questions

Many of the questions in this Study Guide may be representative of the questions which will be used in unit and final examinations by college and university health information management programs. While the content of the questions may also be representative of that tested in the national certifying examinations (discussed in Section Three: How to Prepare for Certification), the question type will be different. Ordinarily, the certifying examinations utilize only multiple choice-type questions and not the variety that is used here or in some colleges and universities for teaching purposes.

Since subject content and its mastery is prerequisite to competent performance as a certified practitioner, this Study Guide includes for your reference the Domains and Subdomains that specify the abilities at entrance into the profession as Registered Health Information Technicians and Registered Health

Information Administrators on the succeeding pages. These statements form the basis for certification examination test construction. Most education programs distribute the current list of competencies to students for reference throughout their coursework. When graduates make application for the certification examination, the test materials mailed to the applicant contain a current list of the competencies to be tested.

## AHIMA Domains and Subdomains

HIM programs are accredited by The Commission on Accreditation of Allied Health Education Programs in collaboration with the Council on Accreditation of the American Health Information Management Association. In order to maintain accreditation, the Program must adhere to the Standards and Guidelines for an Accredited Educational Program for the Health Information Administrator or Health Information Technician. These Standards outline the necessary items for accreditation.

Approximately every two years, the Council on Certification of the American Health Information Management Association (AHIMA) undertakes a job analysis study of the membership, stratified to reflect the entry-level practitioners from the last two years as well as some sample of more experienced practitioners. From this job analysis study, the Council on Certification develops the cognitive domains, and subdomains that will serve as the template for construction of the credentialing examinations. These domains and subdomains are also provided to HIM programs for use in the development and updating of the curriculum, as they identify the current entry-level competencies required of graduates. The current edition of the cognitive domains and subdomains are essential in curriculum development for measuring entry level competence of graduates. The AHIMA Domains and Subdomains are listed below with a chapter guide to *Health Information: Management of a Strategic Resource*, 2nd edition.

## Guide to Domains and Subdomains
## for the Registered Health Information Technician*

| Domains and Subdomains | Chapter(s) in which content is contained in *Health Information: Management of a Strategic Resource, 2ND ed* |
|---|---|
| **I. Domain: Healthcare Data** | |
| **A. Subdomain: Data Structure, Content and Use** | |
| 1. Verify timeliness, completeness, accuracy, and appropriateness of data and data sources (e.g., patient care, management, billing reports and/or databases). | Chapters 3 and 4 |
| 2. Conduct qualitative analysis to assure that documentation in the health record supports the diagnosis and reflects the progress, clinical findings and discharge status. | Chapters 3 and 4 |
| 3. Assist in the facility's billing process. | Chapters 6 and 15 |
| 4. Validate coding accuracy using clinical information found in the health record. | Chapter 6 |
| **B. Subdomain: Clinical Classification Systems—ICD-9-CM Coding** | |
| 1. Assign diagnosis/procedure codes using ICD-9-CM. | Chapter 6 |
| **C. Subdomain: Clinical Classification Systems—CPT Coding** | |
| 1. Assign procedure codes using CPT/HCPCS. | Chapter 6 |
| **II. Domain: Health Information Analysis** | |
| **A. Subdomain: Healthcare Statistics and Research** | |
| 1. Abstract records for department indices/databases/registries. | Chapters 5, 6 and 7 |
| 2. Collect data for quality management, utilization management, risk management, and other patient care related studies. | Chapters 8 and 10 |
| 3. Calculate and interpret healthcare statistics. | Chapter 8 and 9 |
| 4. Present data in verbal and written forms. | Chapters 8 and 9 |

*Adapted with permission from American Health Information Management Association, Chicago, Illinois.

Copyright © 1999 by the American Health Information Management Association. Used with permission.

### B. Subdomain: Clinical Quality Assessment and Performance Improvement

| | |
|---|---|
| 1. Participate in facility-wide quality management program. | Chapter 10 |
| 2. Analyze clinical data to identify trends. | Chapters 8, 9 and 10 |

## III. Domain: Healthcare Environment

### A. Subdomain: Healthcare Delivery Systems

| | |
|---|---|
| 1. Interpret and apply laws, accreditation, licensure and certification standards, monitor changes, and communicate information-related changes to others in the facility. | Chapters 1 and 11 |
| 2. Understand the role of various providers and disciplines throughout the continuum of healthcare services. | Chapters 1 and 2 |

### B. Subdomain: Legal and Ethical Issues

| | |
|---|---|
| 1. Release patient-specific data to authorized users. | Chapter 11 |
| 2. Request patient-specific information from other sources. | Chapter 11 |
| 3. Summarize patient encounter data for release to authorized users. | Chapter 11 |
| 4. Develop policies and procedures to protect unauthorized access to patient records. | Chapter 11 |
| 5. Assist in developing facility-wide confidentiality policies. | Chapter 11 |

### C. Healthcare Information Requirements and Standards

| | |
|---|---|
| 1. Assist in developing health record documentation guidelines. | Chapter 3 |
| 2. Perform quantitative analysis of health records to evaluate compliance with regulations and standards. | Chapter 3 |
| 3. Perform qualitative analysis of health records to evaluate compliance. | Chapter 3 |
| 4. Assist in preparing the facility for an accreditation, licensing and/or certification survey. | Chapters 1, 3, 4, 5 and 10 |
| 5. Develop and demonstrate HIM service compliance with relevant regulations and accreditation standards. | Chapters 3, 4, 5, 6 and 10 |

Copyright © 1999 by the American Health Information Management Association. Used with permission.

|   |   |   |
|---|---|---|
| | 6. Ensure facility-wide adherence to health information services' compliance with regulatory requirements (e.g., ICD-9-CM Cooperating parties coding guidelines, HCFA Compliance Plan, Correct Coding Initiative). | Chapters 3 and 6 |

**IV. Domain: Information Technology & Systems**

    **A. Subdomain: Information Technology**

| | | |
|---|---|---|
| | 1. Use common software packages (e.g., spreadsheets, databases, word processing, graphics, presentation, statistical, e-mail). | Chapters 4 and 16 |
| | 2. Use electronic or imaging technology to store medical records. | Chapters 5 and 17 |
| | 3. Query facility-wide databases to retrieve information. | Chapter 4 |
| | 4. Generate reports from various databases. | Chapters 4, 7, 8 and 9 |
| | 5. Protect data integrity and validity using software or hardware technology. | Chapters 3, 4 and 16 |
| | 6. Enforce confidentiality and security measures to protect electronic information. | Chapters 11 and 16 |
| | 7. Identify common software problems. | Chapters 16 and 17 |
| | 8. Design data quality controls and edits. | Chapters 4 and 18 |
| | 9. Participate in development of strategic and operational plans for facility-wide information systems. | Chapters 12, 13 and 18 |

    **B. Subdomain: Health Information Systems**

| | | |
|---|---|---|
| | 1. Collect and report data on incomplete records and timeliness of record completion. | Chapter 3 |
| | 2. Maintain filing and retrieval systems for paper-based patient records. | Chapter 5 |
| | 3. Maintain integrity of master patient/client index. | Chapter 5 |
| | 4. Maintain integrity of patient numbering and filing systems. | Chapter 5 |
| | 5. Design forms, computer input screens, and other health record documentation tools. | Chapter 4 |
| | 6. Evaluate software packages to determine that they meet user needs. | Chapter 18 |

**V. Domain: Organization and Management**

    **A. Subdomain: Human Resources Management**

| | | |
|---|---|---|
| | 1. Interview prospective employees. | Chapter 14 |

| | | |
|---|---|---|
| 2. | Hire new employees. | Chapter 14 |
| 3. | Develop and implement new staff orientation and training programs. | Chapter 14 |
| 4. | Supervise staff. | Chapter 12 |
| 5. | Collect data on employee performance. | Chapters 13 and 14 |
| 6. | Conduct performance appraisals. | Chapter 14 |
| 7. | Counsel, discipline and terminate staff. | Chapter 14 |
| 8. | Perform job analyses. | Chapter 14 |
| 9. | Develop job descriptions. | Chapter 12 |
| 10. | Conduct in-service education programs on topics related to health information services. | Chapter 14 |
| 11. | Develop and support work teams. | Chapter 13 |

**B. Subdomain: Health Information Services Management**

| | | |
|---|---|---|
| 1. | Monitor staffing levels, turnaround time, productivity and workflow. | Chapter 13 |
| 2. | Assign projects and tasks to appropriate staff. | Chapters 12 and 13 |
| 3. | Develop productivity and control measures. | Chapter 13 |
| 4. | Benchmark staff performance data in relation to department/facility performance standards. | Chapter 13 |
| 5. | Determine resources (equipment and supplies) to meet workload needs. | Chapters 13 and 15 |
| 6. | Develop departmental policies and procedures. | Chapter 12 |
| 7. | Develop strategic plans, goals, and objectives for area of responsibility and communicate to staff. | Chapter 12 |
| 8. | Participate on intradepartmental teams/committees. | Chapter 12 |
| 9. | Participate on facility-wide teams/committees responsible for health information services issues. | Chapter 12 |
| 10. | Coordinate interdepartmental and/or intra-departmental services. | Chapter 13 |
| 11. | Provide consultation, education, and training to users of health information services. | Chapter 14 |
| 12. | Prepare budgets with accompanying justification and monitor adherence. | Chapter 15 |
| 13. | Evaluate effectiveness of department operations and services. | Chapter 13 |

Copyright © 1999 by the American Health Information Management Association. Used with permission.

| | |
|---|---|
| 14. Develop quality control/improvement systems for departmental processes and use quality improvement tools and techniques to improve processes. | Chapter 10 |
| 15. Manage special projects. | Chapter 13 |
| 16. Plan and conduct meetings. | Chapter 14 |
| 17. Resolve customer complaints. | Chapters 13 and 14 |
| 18. Identify departmental resource requirements, determine cost/benefits, communicate requirements to vendors, and evaluate vendor proposals. | Chapters 15 and 18 |
| 19. Assist in redesigning/re-engineering departmental services and operations. | Chapter 13 |
| 20. Prioritize department functions and services. | Chapter 13 |

## Guide to Domains and Subdomains
## for the Registered Health Information Administrator*

| Domains and Subdomains | Chapter(s) in which content is contained in *Health Information: Management of a Strategic Resource*, 2ND ed |
|---|---|
| **I. Domain: Healthcare Data** | |
| **A. Subdomain: Data Structure, Content and Use** | |
| 1. Verify timeliness, completeness, accuracy, and appropriateness of data and data sources (e.g., patient care, management, billing reports and/or databases). | Chapters 3 and 4 |
| 2. Conduct qualitative analysis to assure that documentation in the health record supports the diagnosis and reflects the progress, clinical findings and discharge status. | Chapters 3 and 4 |
| 3. Assist in the facility's billing process. | Chapters 6 and 15 |
| 4. Validate coding accuracy using clinical information found in the health record. | Chapter 6 |
| **B. Subdomain: Clinical Classification Systems—ICD-9-CM Coding** | |
| 1. Assign diagnosis/procedure codes using ICD-9-CM. | Chapter 6 |
| **C. Subdomain: Clinical Classification Systems—CPT Coding** | |
| 1. Assign procedure codes using CPT/HCPCS. | Chapter 6 |
| **II. Domain: Health Information Analysis** | |
| **A. Subdomain: Healthcare Statistics and Research** | |
| 1. Abstract records for department indices/databases/registries. | Chapters 5, 6 and 7 |
| 2. Collect data for quality management, utilization management, risk management, and other patient care related studies. | Chapters 8 and 10 |

*Adapted with permission from American Health Information Management Association, Chicago, Illinois.

Copyright © 1999 by the American Health Information Management Association. Used with permission.

|   |   |   |
|---|---|---|
| | 3. Calculate and interpret healthcare statistics. | Chapters 8 and 9 |
| | 4. Present data in verbal and written forms. | Chapters 8 and 9 |
| **B. Subdomain: Clinical Quality Assessment and Performance Improvement** | | |
| | 1. Participate in facility-wide quality management program. | Chapter 10 |
| | 2. Analyze clinical data to identify trends. | Chapters 8, 9 and 10 |

### III. Domain: Healthcare Environment

#### A. Subdomain: Healthcare Delivery Systems

|   |   |   |
|---|---|---|
| 1. | Interpret and apply laws, accreditation, licensure and certification standards, monitor changes, and communicate information-related changes to others in the facility. | Chapters 1 and 11 |
| 2. | Understand the role of various providers and disciplines throughout the continuum of healthcare services. | Chapters 1 and 2 |

#### B. Subdomain: Legal and Ethical Issues

|   |   |   |
|---|---|---|
| 1. | Release patient-specific data to authorized users. | Chapter 11 |
| 2. | Request patient-specific information from other sources. | Chapter 11 |
| 3. | Summarize patient encounter data for release to authorized users. | Chapter 11 |
| 4. | Develop policies and procedures to protect unauthorized access to patient records. | Chapter 11 |
| 5. | Assist in developing facility-wide confidentiality policies. | Chapter 11 |

#### C. Healthcare Information Requirements and Standards

|   |   |   |
|---|---|---|
| 1. | Assist in developing health record documentation guidelines. | Chapter 3 |
| 2. | Perform quantitative analysis of health records to evaluate compliance with regulations and standards. | Chapter 3 |
| 3. | Perform qualitative analysis of health records to evaluate compliance. | Chapter 3 |
| 4. | Assist in preparing the facility for an accreditation, licensing and/or certification survey. | Chapters 1, 3, 4, 5 and 10 |
| 5. | Develop and demonstrate HIM service compliance with relevant regulations and accreditation standards. | Chapters 3, 4, 5, 6 and 10 |

| | | | |
|---|---|---|---|
| | 6. | Ensure facility-wide adherence to health information services' compliance with regulatory requirements (e.g., ICD-9-CM Cooperating parties coding guidelines, HCFA Compliance Plan, Correct Coding Initiative). | Chapters 3 and 6 |

**IV. Domain: Information Technology & Systems**

    **A. Subdomain: Information Technology**

| | | |
|---|---|---|
| 1. | Use common software packages (e.g., spreadsheets, databases, word processing, graphics, presentation, statistical, e-mail). | Chapters 4 and 16 |
| 2. | Use electronic or imaging technology to store medical records. | Chapters 5 and 17 |
| 3. | Query facility-wide databases to retrieve information. | Chapter 4 |
| 4. | Generate reports from various databases. | Chapters 4, 7, 8 and 9 |
| 5. | Protect data integrity and validity using software or hardware technology. | Chapters 3, 4 and 16 |
| 6. | Enforce confidentiality and security measures to protect electronic information. | Chapters 11 and 16 |
| 7. | Identify common software problems. | Chapters 16 and 17 |
| 8. | Design data quality controls and edits. | Chapters 4 and 18 |
| 9. | Participate in development of strategic and operational plans for facility-wide information systems. | Chapters 12, 13 and 18 |

    **B. Subdomain: Health Information Systems**

| | | |
|---|---|---|
| 1. | Collect and report data on incomplete records and timeliness of record completion. | Chapter 3 |
| 2. | Maintain filing and retrieval systems for paper-based patient records. | Chapter 5 |
| 3. | Maintain integrity of master patient/client index. | Chapter 5 |
| 4. | Maintain integrity of patient numbering and filing systems. | Chapter 5 |
| 5. | Design forms, computer input screens, and other health record documentation tools. | Chapter 4 |
| 6. | Evaluate software packages to determine that they meet user needs. | Chapter 18 |

**V. Domain: Organization and Management**

    **A. Subdomain: Human Resources Management**

| | | |
|---|---|---|
| 1. | Interview prospective employees. | Chapter 14 |

Copyright © 1999 by the American Health Information Management Association. Used with permission.

| | |
|---|---|
| 2. Hire new employees. | Chapter 14 |
| 3. Develop and implement new staff orientation and training programs. | Chapter 14 |
| 4. Supervise staff. | Chapter 12 |
| 5. Collect data on employee performance. | Chapters 13 and 14 |
| 6. Conduct performance appraisals. | Chapter 14 |
| 7. Counsel, discipline and terminate staff. | Chapter 14 |
| 8. Perform job analyses. | Chapter 14 |
| 9. Develop job descriptions. | Chapter 12 |
| 10. Conduct in-service education programs on topics related to health information services. | Chapter 14 |
| 11. Develop and support work teams. | Chapter 13 |
| **B. Subdomain: Health Information Services Management** | |
| 1. Monitor staffing levels, turnaround time, productivity and workflow. | Chapter 13 |
| 2. Assign projects and tasks to appropriate staff. | Chapters 12 and 13 |
| 3. Develop productivity and control measures. | Chapter 13 |
| 4. Benchmark staff performance data in relation to department/facility performance standards. | Chapter 13 |
| 5. Determine resources (equipment and supplies) to meet workload needs. | Chapters 13 and 15 |
| 6. Develop departmental policies and procedures. | Chapter 12 |
| 7. Develop strategic plans, goals, and objectives for area of responsibility and communicate to staff. | Chapter 12 |
| 8. Participate on intradepartmental teams/committees. | Chapter 12 |
| 9. Participate on facility-wide teams/committees responsible for health information services issues. | Chapter 12 |
| 10. Coordinate interdepartmental and/or intra-departmental services. | Chapter 13 |
| 11. Provide consultation, education, and training to users of health information services. | Chapter 14 |
| 12. Prepare budgets with accompanying justification and monitor adherence. | Chapter 15 |
| 13. Evaluate effectiveness of department operations and services. | Chapter 13 |

Copyright © 1999 by the American Health Information Management Association. Used with permission.

| | |
|---|---|
| 14. Develop quality control/improvement systems for departmental processes and use quality improvement tools and techniques to improve processes. | Chapter 10 |
| 15. Manage special projects. | Chapter 13 |
| 16. Plan and conduct meetings. | Chapter 14 |
| 17. Resolve customer complaints. | Chapters 13 and 14 |
| 18. Identify departmental resource requirements, determine cost/benefits, communicate requirements to vendors, and evaluate vendor proposals. | Chapters 15 and 18 |
| 19. Assist in redesigning/re-engineering departmental services and operations. | Chapter 13 |
| 20. Prioritize department functions and services. | Chapter 13 |

Copyright © 1999 by the American Health Information Management Association. Used with permission.

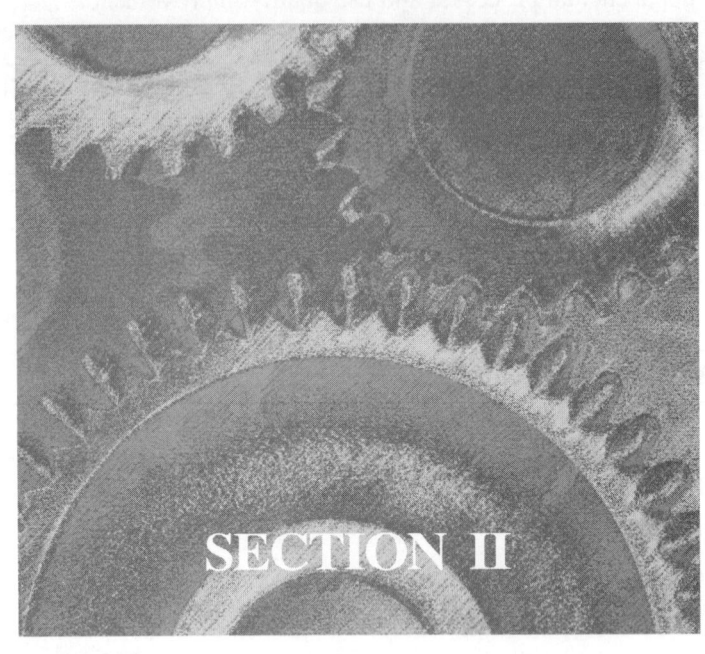

# SECTION II

# REVIEW QUESTIONS AND ASSIGNMENTS BY CHAPTER

# CHAPTER 1

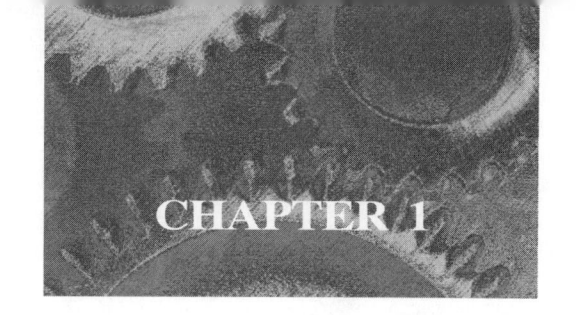

# HEALTH CARE SYSTEMS

## Review

### PRETEST REVIEW

**Directions:**

1. Read each question carefully before selecting an answer.
2. Circle the letter of the correct answer.
3. Answer all the questions since there is no penalty for this pretest review.
4. Check your answers with the answer key located at the end of this chapter.

1. The type of care provided to hospice patients is primarily curative care.
   a. True
   b. False

2. Both state and local governments are responsible for setting objectives for the attainment of goals explicated in the report *Healthy People 2000*.
   a. True
   b. False

3. A completely electronic patient record necessitates the electronic processing of information at the point of service.
   a. True
   b. False

4. The process of measuring a health care facility's compliance with established rules and regulations for Medicare and Medicaid reimbursement is called licensure.
   a. True
   b. False

5. The process of giving legal approval for a health care facility to operate is called certification.
   a. True
   b. False

6. A copayment is a method of direct pay assumed by a subscriber in a managed care setting.
   a. True
   b. False

7. A sliding-scale payment method is commonly employed in managed health care settings.
   a. True
   b. False

8. Native Americans and retired military personnel (including their dependents) are provided health care through CHAMPUS.
   a. True
   b. False

9. When patient average length of stay is greater than 20 days, the facility is classified by the AHA as a long term care facility.
   a. True
   b. False

10. The professional staff organization of a hospital refers to the medical and other credentialed staff (where permitted by state law).
    a. True
    b. False

# CHAPTER REVIEW

## Directions:

1. *Read each question carefully before selecting an answer.*
2. *Circle the letter of the correct answer.*
3. *Answer all the questions since there is no penalty for this pretest review.*
4. *Check your answers with the answer key located at the end of this chapter.*

1. All of the following are true about federal government regulation of health care *except*:
   a. it investigates fraud and abuse arising from any health care facility or licensed physician
   b. it guarantees access to health care
   c. it enacts legislation impacting health care systems
   d. it owns and controls health care facilities

2. All of the following are true about the organizational structure of the DHHS *except*:
   a. the DHHS includes the SSA
   b. the DHHS includes the Office of Inspector General
   c. the DHHS funds and coordinates regional offices
   d. the DHHS established *Healthy People 2000*

3. To be eligible for participation in the Medicare program and for financial reimbursement of its services, health care facilities must demonstrate compliance with the:
   a. *Conditions of Participation*
   b. *Essentials*
   c. standards of the JCAHO
   d. clinical practice guidelines

4. The certification of health care facilities for participation in the Medicare program is the responsibility of the:
   a. federal government
   b. state government
   c. local government
   d. fiscal intermediaries

5. All of the following are true about state government regulation of health care *except*:
   a. it operates public health departments
   b. it administers certification and licensing of health care practitioners
   c. it accredits home health and rehabilitation facilities
   d. it funds medical education through educational institutions

6. Every patient who arrives at a health care facility with an emergency medical condition must be evaluated to determine if the patient condition warrants therapy or transfer to another appropriate health care facility. This was mandated by which legislation?
   a. Occupational Safety and Health Act
   b. Consolidated Omnibus Budget Reconciliation Act
   c. Patient Self-Determination Act
   d. Hill-Burton Act

7. All of the following organizations set voluntary standards for hospitals pertaining to quality health care *except*:
   a. Department of Health and Human Services
   b. American Osteopathic Association
   c. Joint Commission on Accreditation of Health Care Organizations
   d. American College of Surgeons

8. Standards are published by the JCAHO for all of the following types of facilities *except:*
   a. Planned Parenthood organizations
   b. long-term care organizations
   c. non-hospital psychiatric and substance abuse organizations
   d. ambulatory care organizations

9. Which is true of a prospective payment system?
   a. The amount of payment is fixed in advance of services
   b. The amount is based on the provider's statement of cost
   c. It is the designated payment method for all inpatients and outpatients
   d. It is the designated payment according to the patient's ability to pay

10. A reimbursement method that is a prepaid, fixed amount to a provider per each person served is:
    a. direct pay
    b. copayment
    c. capitation
    d. fee-for-service

*Additional review questions can be found on the CD-ROM.*

# Assignments

## 1-1: HEALTH CARE HISTORY AND LEGISLATION

**Assignment:**

*Describe the impact of the following historical events and legislation on health care. How did the health care field change as a result?*

1. Hospital Standardization Program of 1917
2. Hospital Survey and Construction Act of 1946
3. Founding of the Joint Commission on Accreditation of Hospitals in 1952
4. Health Insurance for the Aged Act, Title XVIII of the Social Security Act of 1965
5. Extension of the Kerr-Mills Assistance Program, Title XIX of the Social Security Act of 1965

## 1-2: ACCREDITATION BY THE JOINT COMMISSION ON ACCREDITATION OF HEALTHCARE ORGANIZATIONS (JCAHO)

**Assignment:**

*Utilizing a current JCAHO Accreditation Manual for any of the JCAHO's accreditation programs and the JCAHO's web site www.jcaho.org, respond to the following questions.*

A. List the accreditation programs and the types of facilities accredited by each accreditation program.
B. List and describe the accreditation decisions awarded by the JCAHO.
C. Describe the circumstances when the JCAHO may conduct an unannounced survey.
D. What is the duration of the accreditation awarded?
E. Interpret the scoring scale, i.e. the levels of compliance to the standard. What does each score (1-5) mean?
F. On the JCAHO home page, identify the "audiences" served by this website. List the resources available to each group. Compare and contrast the resources available to each group.

## 1-3: THOUGHT QUESTIONS

**Assignment:**

1. Distinguish between licensure, certification (for Medicare) and accreditation for health care organizations. Define each term. Explain how the three terms are similar and how they are different.
2. Compare the requirements for obtaining licensure as a health care professional, e.g. physician, nurse, to the requirements for obtaining a driver's license by answering the following questions.
   - What steps must a person take to obtain each?
   - What is the purpose of each?
   - Why is the government involved in this process?

Copyright © 2001 by W.B. Saunders Company. All rights reserved.

## 1-4: INTERNET RESOURCES

### Assignment:

*A wealth of information useful to the study of health care systems is available on the Internet. A few of the web sites are listed below and were current at the time of publication.*

### Directions:

1. Select one web site from each category.
2. List the web address and the name of the organization that sponsors the site.
3. Explain the site's primary purpose.
4. Identify the targeted audience.
5. Summarize the content.
6. Briefly outline (list topics) the organization of the information.
7. Print a copy of the home page.
8. Describe how this site would be useful in your professional future.

### Federal Government

Health Care Financing Administration
    www.hcfa.gov

Federal Register
    www.access.gpo.gov/su_docs/aces/aces140.html

National Institute of Health
    www.nih.gov

Center for Disease Control
    www.cdc.gov

### Professional Associations

American Cancer Society
    www.cancer.org

American Medical Association
    www.ama-assn.org

American Hospital Association
    www.aha.org

Rehabilitation Accreditation Commission
    www.carf.org

National League of Nurses
    www.nln.org

**Clinical and Health Information**

Computer Based Patient Record Institute
    www.cpri.org

American Society of Testing and Materials
    www.astm.org

National Library of Medicine
    www.nlm.nih.gov

Agency for Healthcare Research and Quality
    www.ahrq.gov

## 1-5: USING THE AMERICAN HOSPITAL ASSOCIATION (AHA) GUIDE TO THE HEALTH CARE FIELD

### Assignment:

*Utilizing the current* AHA Guide to the Health Care Field, *published by the American Hospital Association, create a table that contains the following information on the 5 largest hospitals and 5 smallest hospitals in your state according to the bed size. For each hospital indicate the:*

- A. Number and type of beds
- B. Hospital ownership: specify if the hospital is governmental vs. nongovernmental, not for profit or proprietary
- C. Clinical specialty or general medical-surgical
- D. Accrediting organization
- E. Population served

## 1-6: HEALTH CARE ORGANIZATIONS/AGENCIES

*Health care services are provided in a variety of settings from preventive screening programs to delivery of "meals on wheels" to the homebound. This exercise will give the opportunity to explore a type of health care organization/agency with which you are not familiar.*

### Assignment:

*Obtain the following information about a local health care organization, excluding acute care hospitals or an agency where you are or have worked or volunteered in the past.*

1. Name of the Organization/Agency
2. Address
3. Contact Person – name, title, credentials
4. List of services offered by the organization/agency (list the services and attach any applicable brochures that describe the agency)
5. Identify where on the continuum of health care these services fit.
6. Identify the owners of the organization/agency and specify whether it is a public, private, not-for-profit, or for-profit organization.
7. Listing and description of the types of organizations with whom the agency is a part of or affiliated. Is it a chapter of a national organization? How does this relationship affect the work of the agency?
8. Description of the types of clients served by the agency, e.g. senior citizens over 55.
9. Source of Funding: Do clients pay for the services? Does any third party reimbursement (insurance) cover the services? Are there limits to the amount of services covered by the payer? Does the agency get funding outside of client fees and reimbursement, e.g., donations, or support from a parent organization?
10. Is the agency licensed? If yes, name the regulations with which the agency must comply. Is the agency accredited? If yes, name the organization and the standards with which this organization must comply.

## 1-7: HEALTH INSURANCE POLICIES

### Assignment:

1. Obtain copies of two different health insurance plans, policies or contracts: One must be for an indemnity plan and one must be for a managed care plan (an HMO, PPO, or POS).
2. Compare and contrast the two insurance plans on all of the following items.
   - benefit
   - benefit period
   - beneficiary
   - co-payments
   - services covered
   - deductible
   - exclusions
   - payer
   - premium
3. Identify which policy would be better for you? Justify your selection.

## 1-8: INSURANCE GRID

### Assignment:

*Complete the grid below by indicating with an X which type of reimbursement mechanism listed across the top with the characteristic listed in the left column.*

| | Characteristic | HMO | PPO | Indemnity Insurance |
|---|---|---|---|---|
| 1. | Capitation | | | |
| 2. | Secondary health care services must be authorized by primary care physician to be paid for (at all) by the third party payer. | | | |
| 3. | Reimbursement will be provided for health care services provided by (any) physician of the patient's choosing. | | | |
| 4. | Fee for service | | | |
| 5. | Choice of primary care physician is limited because payer will not reimburse for services by non-participating physician. | | | |
| 6. | Increased volume of patients for participating providers in turn for discounted charges. | | | |

## 1-9: MEDICARE

## Assignment:

*Using Chapter 1 and the Medicare and You Handbook available in print and on the Internet at http://www.medicare.gov/publications/English.asp, compare and contrast Part A and Part B of Medicare on each of the following dimensions.*

- Eligibility criteria
- Types of health services covered
- Source of funding
- Providers

# Review Answers

## PRETEST REVIEW ANSWER KEY

### Directions:

1. Correct your Pretest answers with the answers below by placing a slash through the incorrect question number (Example: 8) with a pen or pencil of a contrasting color.
2. Record the correct answer by placing a square around the letter of the correct answer.
3. Record the total correct on the Initial Performance Grid in Section 4 of this review manual.
4. Calculate your performance rate and also record on the grid.
5. Promptly locate the correct answer for each question missed in the chapter of the textbook.
6. Proceed to the chapter review if your performance rate was 80% or higher; otherwise, return to the chapter for further study.

### Answers to Pretest Review:

1. b
2. a
3. a
4. b
5. b
6. a
7. b
8. b
9. b
10. a

## CHAPTER REVIEW ANSWER KEY

### Directions:

1. Correct your answers with the answers below by placing a slash through the incorrect question number (Example: 8) with a pen or pencil of a contrasting color.
2. Record the correct answer by placing a square around the letter of the correct answer.
3. Record the total correct on the Initial Performance Grid in Section 4 of this review manual.
4. Calculate your performance rate and also record on the grid.
5. Promptly locate the correct answer for each question missed in the chapter of the textbook.
6. Proceed to the next chapter assigned in your study.

### Answers to Chapter Review:

1. b
2. d
3. a
4. b
5. c
6. b
7. a
8. a
9. a
10. c

Copyright © 2001 by W.B. Saunders Company. All rights reserved.

# CHAPTER 2

# THE HEALTH INFORMATION MANAGEMENT PROFESSION

## Review

### PRETEST REVIEW

**Directions:**

1. Read each question carefully before selecting an answer.
2. Circle the letter of the correct answer.
3. Answer all the questions since there is no penalty for this pretest review.
4. Check your answers with the answer key located at the end of this chapter.

1. The first minimum standards pertaining to the delivery of health care were established by the American Hospital Association.
    a. True
    b. False

2. Early hospital accreditation activities were shared by several organizations including the American Medical Association.
    a. True
    b. False

3. The format of the patient record was significantly changed by the Tax Equity and Fiscal Responsibility Act (TEFRA).
    a. True
    b. False

4. The health record is the source document for verifying claims or bills submitted for reimbursement of care.
    a. True
    b. False

5. The Computer-Based Patient Record Institute (CPRI) is a federal government agency.
    a. True
    b. False

6. AHIMA plays an active role in the development of standards by other organizations such as the JCAHO and ASTM.
    a. True
    b. False

7. The health record is influenced by standards and regulations arising from non-governmental and governmental agencies.
    a. True
    b. False

8. The DRG reimbursement is based on the patient's length of stay and utilization of services.
    a. True
    b. False

9. The *Code of Ethics for Health Information Management* professionals specifically requires one to promote and protect the confidentiality and security of health information.

   a. True
   b. False

10. The involvement of the HIM profession and professional association in the health care reimbursement process was associated with the passage of the Tax Equity and Fiscal Responsibility Act (TEFRA).

    a. True
    b. False

# CHAPTER REVIEW

## Directions:

1. *Read each question carefully before selecting an answer.*
2. *Circle the letter of the correct answer.*
3. *Answer all the questions since there is no penalty for this pretest review.*
4. *Check your answers with the answer key located at the end of this chapter.*

1. Which organization actively demonstrated the need for quality patient records in the early 1900s?.
   a. ACS
   b. AHA
   c. AMRA
   d. JCAH

2. The *Conditions of Participation* are required federal standards for hospitals to follow whether or not they serve Medicare patients.
   a. True
   b. False

3. The DRG system applies to inpatient hospital services which are reimbursed by Medicare.
   a. True
   b. False

4. The Health Insurance Portability and Accountability Act (HIPAA) established requirements for national security standards to protect health care information maintained in electronic data bases.
   a. True
   b. False

5. The AHIMA collaborates with the CAAHEP to accredit academic programs in health information technology and health information administration.
   a. True
   b. False

6. Utilization of services and the quality of care rendered to Medicare patients are monitored by internal review constituencies on behalf of HCFA.
   a. True
   b. False

7. Capitated care was a step toward changing the incentives in health care.
   a. True
   b. False

8. What was the name given to the initial organization currently named AHIMA?
   a. Association of Record Librarians of North America
   b. American Association of Record Librarians
   c. Association of Medical Record Clerks
   d. American Association of Medical Record Workers

9. Compliance with JCAHO standards is voluntary for health care organizations.
   a. True
   b. False

10. Consumer "report cards" on the performance of health care organizations are derived from data extracted from individual patient records and billing reports and then aggregated for public reporting.
    a. True
    b. False

*Additional review questions can be found on the CD-ROM.*

# Assignments

## 2-1: AHIMA WEB SITE

### Assignment:

*This assignment will introduce you to the resources of the American Health Information Management Association, its Component State Associations and its allied associations through the WWW. (The web address and settings were current at the time of publication.)*

### Directions:

1. Access http://www.ahima.org and from the AHIMA Home Page, select <About AHIMA>.
   A. Locate "Members in the Workplace" to find:
      i. The types of functions that HIM professionals are uniquely educated to perform within health care organizations.
      ii. List the types of organizations in which AHIMA members work in addition to "hospitals".
   B. Click on the "AHIMA History" information available on the Website and list the 3 names this Association has had over the years.
   C. Click on the "AHIMA Mission" and describe the purpose of the AHIMA.
   D. Click on "AHIMA Bylaws", and specifically review the following sections of the Bylaws to answer the question(s) below:
      i. Membership – What are the membership categories?
      ii. House of Delegates – What is its purpose? Who are its members?
      iii. Councils – Name the councils, describe how its members are chosen and explain the purpose of each council.
      iv. Committees – Name the standing committees and explain the purpose of each.
2. Return to the AHIMA Home Page (http://ww.ahima.org) and select <Careers>, and create a grid to compare the of health information administrators, health information technicians and coding specialists using the following categories:
   A. requirements for education
   B. certification titles
   C. continuing education requirements
3. Return to the AHIMA Home Page (http://www.ahima.org) and select <Specialty Groups>.
   A. List the specialty groups which currently exist within AHIMA.
   B. Select one specialty group and read about it: print the information about the specialty group you visit and attach to this report.
4. Return to the AHIMA Home Page (http://www.ahima.org) and select <State Associations>:
   A. Select a state from the list of CSAs, print and attach the information available about that state association to this report. Note: if the state has a website, visit their website as well and identify job openings posted on the website that would be of interest to you.

5. Return to the AHIMA Home Page (http://www.ahima.org) and select <FORE>.
   A. Select "FORE Library" and describe how it relates to the National Information Center on Health Services Administration.
   B. Select "Scholarships and Loans" and describe who is eligible to apply for scholarship and/or loan support through FORE.
6. Leave the AHIMA website and visit http://www.jhita.org:
   A. Describe the purpose or mission of the Joint Health Information and Technology Alliance (JHITA).
   B. List the names of the member organizations of JHITA.
   C. Select one of the member organizations (not AHIMA) and visit its website, then briefly describe who this specific organization represents or serves.

## 2-2: JCAHO RESOURCES

### Assignment:

*This exercise will introduce you to the timely resources provided via the World Wide Web (WWW) specifically to the resources of the Joint Commission on Accreditation of Healthcare Organizations (JCAHO).*

### Directions:

1. At the JCAHO home page http://www.jcaho.org, select the following links to get to "Joint Commission Perspectives" newsletter.
   - "Education and Publications",
   - "Newsletters and Journals"
   - <show me> next to "Joint Commission Perspectives"
   - "Review a Sample Issue":
     1) Select and read one (1) article in the sample Perspectives issue
     2) Write a summary of the key points communicated by the article
2. Return to the JCAHO Home Page, visit another section of your choice and describe in writing what you discovered during this visit.

## 2-3: TOUR OF A HEALTH INFORMATION SERVICES DEPARTMENT

### Tour Objectives for Tour Guide and Students:

- Describe the organizational structure of the department, including an identification of which positions within the department are occupied by various types of credentialed HIM professionals: RHIA, RHIT, and CCS.
- Identify and briefly describe the various functions which constitute the work of the health information services department.
- Briefly explain the work flow within the department.
- Discuss who the "customers" of the department are and what their basic expectations are with respect to quality service from the department.

### Directions:

*At the conclusion of the tour, prepare a reflective essay entitled: HIM Services: Behind the Scenes of Patient Care – by <Your Name> focusing on the knowledge and insights gained from this experience.*

## 2-4: HIM ETHICS

## Assignment:

*For each of the following situations and based on the AHIMA Code of Ethics:*

1. Determine if the health information management professional (HIM) acted ethically or unethically.
2. If unethically, describe why the action was unethical.
3. Describe how the situation should have been handled in an ethical manner.

| Situation | Ethical/Unethical | Ethical Behavior |
|---|---|---|
| 1. HIM receives a call from a friend who asks whether or not she should consult with Dr. Doe who is on the staff of the hospital. HIM replies, "Heavens no, he doesn't have many cases at the hospital, and his patients have a lot of complications after their surgery. You'd better go to Dr. Roe, he's wonderful." | | |
| 2. At her exercise class, one of the members of the class expresses sympathy for an absent member who, she reports, has recently been hospitalized because of acute appendicitis. HIM remarks, "It wasn't appendicitis at all, but of course, I can't tell you what it was because that wouldn't be ethical." | | |
| 3. A patient's record has been subpoenaed for production in court. HIM appears at court with the record, but has not been called to testify when the noon recess is called. The attorney who subpoenaed the record, and who has been unable to secure the patient's permission to review it, invites HIM to lunch. During lunch the attorney asks HIM to see the record, explaining that he will get the information anyhow once she testifies. If he gets to see it now, time will be saved and justice expedited. HIM agrees and lets the attorney see the record. | | |

4. HIM is employed as a Director of Health Information Management at the Community Hospital. HIM has decided to teach medical terminology at the local Community College. HIM is being paid for teaching this course plus her salary from the hospital. HIM told her boss that she would be unavailable on Tuesday night because of her commitment to teach this course.

5. An inexperienced person has been employed to manage the health information department at a small neighboring clinic. This person asks HIM for advice. HIM, believing that he has more than enough to do taking care of his own work, tells this person that he cannot help her.

6. Dr. Smith has re-dictated a history and physical exam report on a patient who was discharged two months ago. The new report states that the patient had a back injury due to an auto accident. The original report referred to the condition as chronic back pain. HIM complies with the doctor's request and files the new report in the patient's record and removes the old one. After all, the doctor is always right.

7. When applying for a fellowship in the American College of Surgeons, Dr. X uses, as examples of his own surgical work, the cases of several patients who were actually cared for by a senior surgeon on the staff. When the list of cases he has submitted is sent to the hospital for verification, HIM, knowing how anxious he is to obtain this qualification and not wanting to make trouble, verifies by signature the statements that these were Dr. X's patients.

8. Returning from a meeting of the Surgical Case Review Committee, where he took minutes, HIM excitedly informs his assistant, "You know Dr. Blank, the one who's so ugly about completing her records—well, they said today that the big operation she did last month on Mary Jones was not necessary at all. They're recommending that her surgical privileges be suspended!"

9. A bill is returned from the fiscal intermediary with a letter requesting copies of records to justify the diagnosis and treatment. The code numbers that appear on the bill are different from those on the patient's record. Upon checking, HIM finds that the codes on the bill put the case into a higher paying DRG and the documentation in the patient record does not justify the new codes. HIM decides to send portions of the record and not change the codes to see if the FI catches the discrepancy.

10. HIM begins working at a small rural hospital. He has a personal computer in his office and would like to use it for statistical reports and graphics. The administrator offers a copy of a spreadsheet software package that she uses. The administrator refuses to purchase another copy for HIM when the hospital already owns one. HIM installs the same software on his computer in the HIM department.

# Review Answers

## PRETEST REVIEW ANSWER KEY

### Directions:

1. Correct your Pretest answers with the answers below by placing a slash through the incorrect question number (Example: 8) with a pen or pencil of a contrasting color.
2. Record the correct answer by placing a square around the letter of the correct answer.
3. Record the total correct on the Initial Performance Grid in Section 4 of this review manual.
4. Calculate your performance rate and also record on the grid.
5. Promptly locate the correct answer for each question missed in the chapter of the textbook.
6. Proceed to the chapter review if your performance rate was 80% or higher; otherwise, return to the chapter for further study.

### Answers to Pretest Review:

| 1. | b | 6.  | a |
|----|---|-----|---|
| 2. | a | 7.  | a |
| 3. | b | 8.  | b |
| 4. | a | 9.  | a |
| 5. | b | 10. | a |

## CHAPTER REVIEW ANSWER KEY

### Directions:

1. Correct your answers with the answers below by placing a slash through the incorrect question number (Example: 8) with a pen or pencil of a contrasting color.
2. Record the correct answer by placing a square around the letter of the correct answer.
3. Record the total correct on the Initial Performance Grid in Section 4 of this review manual.
4. Calculate your performance rate and also record on the grid.
5. Promptly locate the correct answer for each question missed in the chapter of the textbook.
6. Proceed to the next chapter assigned in your study.

### Answers to Chapter Review:

| 1. | a | 6.  | b |
|----|---|-----|---|
| 2. | b | 7.  | a |
| 3. | a | 8.  | a |
| 4. | a | 9.  | a |
| 5. | a | 10. | a |

Copyright © 2001 by W.B. Saunders Company. All rights reserved.

# CHAPTER 3

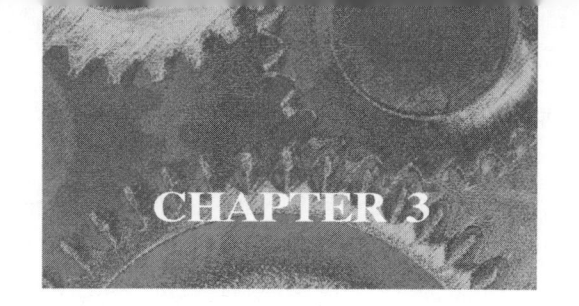

# DATA COLLECTION STANDARDS

## Review

**PRETEST REVIEW**

### Directions:

1. Read each question carefully before selecting an answer.
2. Circle the letter of the correct answer.
3. Answer all the questions since there is no penalty for this pretest review.
4. Check your answers with the answer key located at the end of this chapter.

1. Standards formulated by agencies called practice guidelines are not enforceable.
   a. True
   b. False

2. Diagnostic and procedure indexes are a source of primary data.
   a. True
   b. False

3. Utilization review personnel collect data relative to a facility's efficiency.
   a. True
   b. False

4. The UHDDS was first developed by the JCAHO.
   a. True
   b. False

5. Data sets standardize both the data collected and the information reported for comparative purposes.
   a. True
   b. False

6. The Omnibus Reconciliation Act of 1987 mandated the use of the Minimum Data Set for long term-care.
   a. True
   b. False

7. PROs are required to evaluate the quality of care provided to hospital inpatients and outpatients.
   a. True
   b. False

8. The extent to which data meet the goals and needs of an organization refers to its appropriateness.
   a. True
   b. False

9. The Resident Assessment Protocol is part of the Minimum Data Set for use in long-term care.
   a. True
   b. False

10. Data have reliability when they are meaningful and relevant to their stated purpose.
    a. True
    b. False

# CHAPTER REVIEW

## Directions:

1. *Read each question carefully before selecting an answer.*
2. *Circle the letter of the correct answer.*
3. *Answer all the questions since there is no penalty for this pretest review.*
4. *Check your answers with the answer key located at the end of this chapter.*

1. All of the following are data elements included in the MDS *except:*
   a. cognition
   b. daily patterns of activity
   c. principal procedure
   d. psychosocial status

2. The judicial process uses _____ to settle an injury case involving an automobile accident.
   a. aggregate data
   b. primary data
   c. case mix data
   d. registry data

3. Blue Cross/Blue Shield uses _____ to resolve a claim for payment.
   a. primary data
   b. case mix data
   c. both a and b
   d. neither a nor b

4. Patients use _____ to research their genetic history.
   a. primary data
   b. case mix data
   c. registry data
   d. secondary data

5. Which organization does not promulgate standards or regulations relating to data quality management?
   a. AHIMA
   b. HCFA
   c. PPO
   d. JCAHO

6. Which is a software program for tracking the utilization of services in managed care settings?
   a. Ambulatory Care Group Case Mix Management System
   b. Clinical Information Management System
   c. Uniform Clinical Data Set
   d. Uniform Ambulatory Care Data Set

7. The term "demographics" is often used in reference to what type of data?
   a. financial
   b. socioeconomic
   c. clinical
   d. primary

8. Which of the following collects discharge data on federally-funded patients?
   a. Minimum Data Set
   b. National Practitioner Data Bank
   c. Resident Assessment Protocol
   d. Uniform Hospital Discharge Data Set

---

### DISCHARGE SUMMARY

Patient: Peter N. Smith         00-14-92         Room: 316.2

This 50-year-old man was admitted to the hospital on December 29, 1991, in a state of acute hyperactivity. He laughed and joked freely, exhibited flight of ideas, with no evidence of hallucinations or delusions. He has had a history of previous similar episodes dating back to 1963.

He was treated with electric shock therapy and phenothiazines, gradually improved and after eight shock treatments appeared dull, vacant, and confused. He was then switched to sleep therapy with sodium amytal, remained confused for the next several days. Gradually his memory improved. Then his mood became one of depression. This was treated with psychotherapy and antidepressant medications. He was discharged on January 26, 1992.

Final diagnosis: Manic-depressive illness, manic phase.

_____

John James, M.D.

---

Questions 9, 10, 11:

Referring to the discharge summary above, identify general data elements missing from the report which are required by the JCAHO standards. Do not include the fact that the summary was not signed.

*Additional review questions can be found on the CD-ROM.*

# Assignments

## 3-1: INTERNAL DATA SOURCES

**Assignment:**

*Identify the data elements collected by the following health care providers:*

- Physicians
- Nursing Personnel
- Ancillary Departments
- Administration

## 3-2: EXTERNAL DATA NEEDS OF A HEALTH CARE ORGANIZATION

**Assignment:**

*Health Care Organizations generate a lot of data and information but they also need data and information to remain competitive in their environments. Identify the types of data needed by a health care organization about its external environment to remain competitive and viable.*

## 3-3: USERS OF HEALTH CARE DATA

**Assignment:**

*Explain how each of the following groups use health care data.*

- Providers
- Payers
- Employers
- Governmental Agencies
- Patients

## 3-4: ROLE OF THE HEALTH INFORMATION MANAGER

### Assignment:

*Prepare an oral report for presentation to the group on the role of the Health Information Management Professional in the collection and use of data in one of the settings listed below. Each student will report on a different type of organization. The presentation will be a minimum of 15 minutes in length and will require the use of handout materials, audiovisual software, or posters to highlight key points in the discussion.*

- A. Acute care hospital
- B. Long term care facility
- C. Home care agency
- D. Health maintenance organization
- E. Cancer registry
- F. Emergency medical care
- G. Outpatient surgical center
- H. Outpatient clinic/physicians' private practice

Grades will be based on the following criteria:
1. Quality—completeness and accuracy—of information
2. Quality of presentation
    - A. proper use of grammar, etc.
    - B. voice: projection, volume and pace
    - C. eye contact, gestures
    - D. ability to answer questions
3. Quality of handouts and audiovisuals
    - A. clarity
    - B. readability
    - C. pertinence to presentation
4. Effective use of time

## 3-5: UNIFORM HOSPITAL DISCHARGE DATA SET (UHDDS)

## Assignment:

1. Describe the types of data that are classified as:
   Socioeconomic
   Financial
   Clinical

2. Using an inpatient acute care hospital record and the attached worksheet, identify each element of the UHDDS present within the record. For each element, identify the data from the patient record. Classify each of the UHDDS elements as either socioeconomic, financial or clinical. Refer to Chapter 3: Data Collection Standards for explanation of the elements of the UHDDS.

3. Review the record to determine if it appears to have been completed in a timely way. Are all aspects timely? Identify those that are and those that are not. Support your statements with factual data.

4. Review the record to determine if it is accurate and complete. Support your statements with factual data.

## 3-5: WORKSHEET: UNIFORM HOSPITAL DISCHARGE DATA SET (UHDDS)

| Data Element | Data Found In Record | Classification Of Data (Socioeconomic, Financial, Clinical |
|---|---|---|
| Personal identification | | |
| Date of Birth | | |
| Sex | | |
| Race and Ethnicity | | |
| Residence | | |
| Hospital Identification | | |
| Admission Date | | |
| Type of Admission (scheduled/unscheduled) | | |
| Discharge Date | | |
| Attending physician ID | | |
| Operating physician ID | | |
| Principal Diagnosis | | |
| Other Diagnoses | | |
| Qualifier for Other Diagnoses | | |
| External Cause of Injury Code | | |
| Procedure and Dates | | |
| Disposition of Patient | | |
| Patient's Expected Source of Payment: Primary and Other | | |
| Total Charges | | |

## 3-6: PATIENT RECORD CONTENT

## Assignment:

1. Select two reports from a patient record, e.g., face sheet, history and physical exam report, operative report, etc.
2. Using the worksheet below, classify data items from the report by ASTM E1384 categories and data elements.

**ASTM E1384 Worksheet**
**Report Title:**

| Data Element | E1384 Category | E1384 Data Element |
|---|---|---|
| 1. | | |
| 2. | | |
| 3. | | |
| 4. | | |
| 5. | | |
| 6. | | |
| 7. | | |
| 8. | | |
| 9. | | |
| 10. | | |
| 11. | | |
| 12. | | |
| 13. | | |
| 14. | | |
| 15. | | |

Copyright © 2001 by W.B. Saunders Company. All rights reserved.

## 3-7: COLLECTION OF HEALTH CARE DATA ACROSS THE HEALTH CARE CONTINUUM

### Assignment:

1. For each of the following five major types of health care delivery systems, identify the data collection issues.
2. Compare and contrast the issues for each system.
    - Ambulatory Care
    - Acute Care
    - Home Care (including hospice)
    - Long Term Care (including rehabilitation)
    - Mental Health Care

## 3-8: DOCUMENTATION ANALYSIS IN NON-ACUTE CARE HOSPITAL SETTINGS

### Assignment:

*For the assigned type of health care facility, prepare a 20-minute presentation that includes at least:*

1. The process of obtaining input of data into both paper and electronic health record systems,
2. The method(s) used to assure that information is present and authenticated. Description of the method(s) should include sample forms/screens and written procedures,
3. The qualifications and/or training of the individual(s) who perform(s) the reviews, (a job description),
4. Other activities that are performed in conjunction with the reviews (e.g., performed concurrently with coding and abstracting, record assembly, etc.),
5. The percentage of records on which the review is performed (all or a sample—if a sample, how are the records selected?),
6. Frequency of reviews,
7. Are Quality Improvement (QI) studies performed to assess the quality of the content of the documents? If yes, list the criteria or include a worksheet used for the study,
8. Any other information that would be useful to understand the process,
9. Resources: books and journal articles, and HIM directors at the health care settings.

Evaluation of the presentation will be based on the completeness of the information given and the professionalism of the presentation. Use of handouts, audiovisual software (large print), or other appropriate teaching tools is recommended.

### Topics: (Each student or group of students will do a different topic.)

1. Nursing facility (long-term care)
2. Mental retardation/developmental disability facility
3. Hospice
4. Physicians' group practice (10 doctors or more)
5. Free standing outpatient surgical center
6. Home health agency

7. Mental (behavioral) health facility
8. Chemical dependency treatment facility
9. Teaching hospital outpatient clinic
10. Correctional facility – health care unit
11. Rehabilitation facility
12. Emergicenter or urgent care center

## 3-9: EVALUATION OF CONTENT OF AN INPATIENT ACUTE CARE HOSPITAL RECORD

### Assignment:

*Respond to the questions below to evaluate the content of a patient record to determine if it meets the JCAHO requirements.*

### Materials needed:

1. A hospital inpatient record.
2. *Comprehensive Accreditation Manual for Hospitals.* Chicago, Joint Commission on Healthcare Organizations, latest edition. Refer especially to section IM7, Patient-Specific Data/Information

### Questions:

1. History and Physical

    Does the H & P include the items required by the JCAHO? If not, what is missing? Is there an interval note if needed?

    What are the time requirements for completion of an H&P? Interval note?

    Does the record meet these deadlines?

2. Physician Orders

    What are the JCAHO time requirements for signatures/authentication of physician verbal orders?

    Verbal/Telephone orders:
    - If present, are the verbal orders on the record signed/authenticated?
    - Can you determine when they were signed/authenticated by the physician?
    - Assume that the hospital has a requirement that verbal/telephone orders must be signed within 48 hours; does the record meet this requirement? How can you tell?

    Standing orders:
    - What are standing orders?
    - Identify any standing orders within your record.
    - How do they differ from other orders?

3. Consents
    - Does the record include a signed consent for treatment?
    - Is it signed?
    - What is the relationship of the person who signed it to the patient?
    - Was it signed prior to treatment?
    - Besides the consent form does the record contain evidence that indicates the procedure was discussed with the patient and that he/she understood?
    - What other consent/authorization forms are present in the record?
    - Are they signed by the patient/patient's legal representative?

4. Physician progress notes
   - Do the physicians' progress notes on the record follow the JCAHO recommended standards for timeliness and completeness?
   - Explain how by citing specific examples documented in the record to illustrate your evaluation.
5. Laboratory/radiology reports
   - Is there a laboratory or radiology report for every physician's order for a lab or radiology exam?
   - Are there any lab or x-ray tests present for which there are no physician's order?
   - If yes to either of the two previous questions, describe the differences.
6. Operative Report
   - Does the pre-op diagnosis on the operative report agree with the provisional diagnosis or impression on the admitting history and physical exam report? Post-op diagnosis?
   - Does the operative report contain the required elements? If no, list the missing items.
7. Pathology Report
   - Was any tissue removed at surgery? If yes, is the pathology report in the record?
   - Is the pathology diagnosis consistent with the postoperative diagnosis?
8. Anesthesia Report
   - Does the record include pre-operative and post-operative anesthesia information? Where is it located?
   - What does the pre-anesthesia evaluation indicate about this patient? Is it complete?
   - Evaluate the legibility of the information.
   - What further references or additional forms in this record would be helpful to interpret the data?
9. Clinical Resume/Physician's Discharge Summary
   - Identify the types of patients for which the JCAHO requires a discharge summary.
   - Does your record require a discharge summary? Why or why not?
   - Does the discharge summary meet the JCAHO requirements? If it does not, what items are missing?
   - What is the difference between the detailed discharge summary and the face sheet?
   - What is included on the discharge summary that is not on the face sheet and vice versa?
10. Computer forms
    - List the titles of all documents in the record that were prepared by or completed on a computer (other than transcribed reports).

*The original project concept was based on an assignment developed by Kathleen Waters, M.Ed., RHIA, Professor in the Health Information Administration Program, University of Washington, Seattle. Revised by Donna Wilde, MPA, RHIA.*

64 ■ Study Guide to Accompany Health Information: Management of a Strategic Resource

## 3-10: ONGOING RECORD REVIEW

### Assignment:

*At the JCAHO website, obtain copies of the Medical Record Review Tool and use it to evaluate medical records.*

### Directions:

1. At the JCAHO website (www.jcaho.org), select "Health Care Organizations and Professionals" section; and then scroll and select "Medical Record Review".
2. Print off copies of the Medical Record Review Tool – Part I and II.
3. Evaluate records provided by the instructor using this tool.
4. Create tables and graphs showing the results of your review.

## 3-11: DELINQUENT RECORD STATISTICS

### Case Study:

The hospital is due for a JCAHO accreditation survey in six months. The CEO asks for a report regarding the medical staff's compliance with the JCAHO requirements for delinquent records for last year. He wishes to avoid a Type 1 citation related to numbers of delinquent records.

### Directions:

1. Input the data found on the following page into a computerized spreadsheet program.
2. Using the spreadsheet software, calculate the total number of discharges for the month. For purposes of delinquent record calculations, add the total inpatient discharges to the total ambulatory surgeries for each month.
3. Place totals for the year in the total column for the first five rows.
4. Have the computer calculate and insert the number of delinquent records, history and physical exam reports (H & Ps), and operative reports permitted by the JCAHO for each month in 200x based on the hospital's statistics for that month (i.e., the sum of the inpatient discharges and outpatient surgeries that month should be the denominator for the calculation of delinquent records and H & Ps). Refer to the JCAHO Scoring Guidelines and text for delinquent record requirements (e.g. avoid a Type 1 citation). To calculate the year's figures, the monthly average should be used. Therefore, add a final monthly average column and have the computer compute the averages for all rows.
5. Using the spreadsheet's graphics options, construct both a line graph and a bar graph showing the hospital's total number of delinquent records as compared to the total number of delinquent records allowed by JCAHO for the twelve months in 200X (do not include the total for the year). Which of the above two graphs do you prefer in illustrating the hospital's compliance? Why?
6. Provide a narrative analysis of the findings for the hospital CEO. Reference the table and graphs in the report. Include in the analysis whether the hospital was in compliance with JCAHO standards in each of the three areas during each month of the year. Was the hospital in compliance for the whole year?

Copyright © 2001 by W.B. Saunders Company. All rights reserved.

*Northern Expanse Hospital*
*Polar, Alaska*
*Delinquent Record Report—200X*

| Item | Jan | Feb | Mar | Apr | May | June | Jul | Aug | Sep | Oct | Nov | Dec | Total |
|---|---|---|---|---|---|---|---|---|---|---|---|---|---|
| Total Inpatient Discharges | 1499 | 1311 | 1297 | 1314 | 1708 | 1567 | 1736 | 1499 | 1578 | 1609 | 1588 | 1834 | |
| Total Ambulatory Surgeries | 168 | 243 | 289 | 348 | 551 | 296 | 342 | 350 | 301 | 333 | 312 | 421 | |
| Total Inpatient Operations | 672 | 888 | 553 | 540 | 354 | 468 | 494 | 416 | 518 | 437 | 279 | 599 | |
| Total Discharges | | | | | | | | | | | | | |
| Total Operations | | | | | | | | | | | | | |
| Actual Delinquent Records | 426 | 391 | 406 | 429 | 509 | 614 | 598 | 679 | 796 | 690 | 537 | 711 | |
| Actual Delinquent H & Ps | 27 | 15 | 31 | 7 | 23 | 21 | 18 | 9 | 11 | 34 | 46 | 39 | |
| Actual Delinquent Operative Reports | 13 | 14 | 20 | 18 | 26 | 30 | 29 | 37 | 42 | 59 | 33 | 34 | |
| Number of Delinquent Records Permitted | | | | | | | | | | | | | |
| Number of Delinquent H & Ps Permitted | | | | | | | | | | | | | |
| Number of Delinquent Operative Reports Permitted | | | | | | | | | | | | | |

## 3-12: PHYSICIAN INTERVIEWS

*Physicians are the primary users of patient information. These interviews will provide the opportunity to speak with physicians and discover their needs and preferences for information.*

### Directions:

1. Interview five physicians to obtain information regarding their routine information needs and preferences in their practices.
2. Summarize the responses in a narrative report. Analyze the results for their impact on development of an electronic health record system for a physician's practice.
3. If practical, share and compare the interview results with classmates.

The interview responses must address all of the following:

1. Name of physician, specialty, location of office, number of physicians in the practice, number of offices, hospital affiliations (specify medical staff category, e.g., active, consulting, for each affiliation). What percent of the practice is inpatient, acute care, long term care, home health care, etc.? What percent is outpatient?
2. Using the list below, identify the type of information the physicians find most helpful in caring for their patients. Do they experience any difficulties in getting access to this information? If there are problems in obtaining the information, what do they consider to be the cause of the problems?
    A. Medications. What time period, e.g., medications on inpatient discharge?
    B. Lab values. Which ones? What time frame, e.g., during the last year only, or for all time?
    C. Pathology. Whole report, or diagnosis only?
    D. Radiology. Whole report, or diagnosis only?
    E. Other diagnostic exams. Which ones are most helpful? Whole report or just results?
    F. Diagnoses. Principle, secondary? Problem lists?
    G. Procedures. Those done by physicians only or others (e.g., speech therapy)?
    H. Alerts. What kind, e.g., allergies, etc.?
    I. Nursing records. Which ones?
    J. Clinic/office notes? All? The most recent? How far back in time are these routinely reviewed?
    K. History and physical examination?
    L. Discharge summary?
    M. Other?
3. Do the physicians currently use computers in their practice? Do they use a computer workstation with access to their clinic/office database? If they have more than one office, are the information systems connected? If yes, how? Do they have access to the hospital information system? If yes, what information do they obtain from it? How frequently? Do they have staff members locate the information for them?
4. Where is the preferred location for computer terminals —in the exam room? In their private office? In an area near the exam rooms? At the bedside in an inpatient facility? Nursing station?

5. What is the preferred format for the record? All on computer, some on computer, some on paper? If some on paper, what portions?
6. Do the physicians need training in computer use? Do they feel comfortable using computers?

## 3-13: OCCUPATIONAL HEALTH RECORDS

### Case Study:

Company officials at a new large manufacturing plant have decided to set up an on-site outpatient medical clinic. The clinic will provide care for injured or ill employees and new and annual employee physicals. They will also perform routine periodic blood and urine tests on their workers since employees will be working around hazardous materials. All services will be free to the employees (the company picking up the expenses).

You have been hired as the Health Information Manager and know nothing about occupational health records.

### Directions:

1. Identify five resources or references that could be consulted to determine the requirements for health data and health information systems for an occupational health center. Use a variety of books, journals or outside resources or individuals to investigate the answer.

   Use a standard bibliographical format to cite references. Describe the content of each reference in a paragraph justifying its usefulness for this setting. Include the names and titles of individuals contacted regarding this assignment.

2. List the types of information needed in an occupational health record. Do not list data item requirements, just the general categories of information.

## 3-14: THOUGHT QUESTIONS

### Assignment:

*Answer the following questions in narrative style. Use information from the text, class discussions, literature review, life experience, and/or discussions with current HIM practitioners.*

1. List criteria to be used for a quality improvement (QI) study on the quality of documentation on a history and physical. Describe the methods to select the sample of records.
2. Contact five health information management professionals or consultants who work in long-term care. Obtain the titles of the QI studies on documentation they completed during the past 12 months.
3. Explain how record completeness and accuracy relates to reimbursement for the patient's care?
4. Review the roles of the HIM manager. How can HIM professionals market their services to facility administrators, physicians, and staff?
5. Do prison health records have data and record form/format standards in your state? Does this help or hinder data quality? Why?

# Review Answers

## PRETEST REVIEW ANSWER KEY

### Directions:

1. Correct your Pretest answers with the answers below by placing a slash through the incorrect question number (Example: 8̸) with a pen or pencil of a contrasting color.
2. Record the correct answer by placing a square around the letter of the correct answer.
3. Record the total correct on the Initial Performance Grid in Section 4 of this review manual.
4. Calculate your performance rate and also record on the grid.
5. Promptly locate the correct answer for each question missed in the chapter of the textbook.
6. Proceed to the chapter review if your performance rate was 80% or higher; otherwise, return to the chapter for further study.

### Answers to Pretest Review:

1. a
2. b
3. a
4. b
5. a
6. a
7. b
8. a
9. b
10. b

## CHAPTER REVIEW ANSWER KEY

### Directions:

1. Correct your answers with the answers below by placing a slash through the incorrect question number (Example: 8̸) with a pen or pencil of a contrasting color.
2. Record the correct answer by placing a square around the letter of the correct answer.
3. Record the total correct on the Initial Performance Grid in Section 4 of this review manual.
4. Calculate your performance rate and also record on the grid.
5. Promptly locate the correct answer for each question missed in the chapter of the textbook.
6. Proceed to the next chapter assigned in your study.

### Answers to Chapter Review:

1. c
2. b
3. c
4. a
5. c
6. a
7. b
8. d
9. significant findings
10. patient's condition on discharge
11. instructions to patient/family

Copyright © 2001 by W.B. Saunders Company. All rights reserved.

# CHAPTER 4

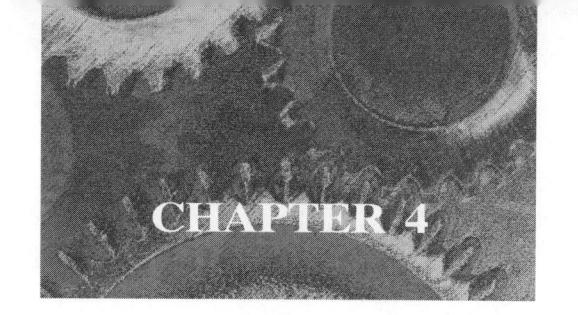

# DATA QUALITY AND TECHNOLOGY

## Review

### PRETEST REVIEW

### Directions:

1. Read each question carefully before selecting an answer.
2. Circle the letter of the correct answer.
3. Answer all the questions since there is no penalty for this pretest review.
4. Check your answers with the answer key located at the end of this chapter.

1. A computer validation check can identify unreasonable values in a given circumstance, such as an unreasonably high laboratory value that would have a zero chance of ever occurring.
    a. True
    b. False

2. Graphical user interfaces control data output.
    a. True
    b. False

3. Audit trails ensure the processing of all items by adding numbers in a specific data field.
    a. True
    b. False

4. Testing the "restore" capabilities of a system is a mechanism for verifying backup system ability.
    a. True
    b. False

5. The storage and retrieval of information from a database is accomplished by a database management system.
    a. True
    b. False

6. ICD-9-CM codes are classified as a "numerical" type of field in a database.
    a. True
    b. False

7. Date, time, and logic are types of fields in a database.
    a. True
    b. False

8. Narrative information can be a type of data field used in a database.
    a. True
    b. False

9. Another term for "data field" is "column."
   a. True
   b. False

10. All the data in a computerized database about patient Morgan Williamson is called a _____.
    a. file
    b. record

# CHAPTER REVIEW

## Directions:

1. *Read each question carefully before selecting an answer.*
2. *Circle the letter of the correct answer.*
3. *Answer all the questions since there is no penalty for this pretest review.*
4. *Check your answers with the answer key located at the end of this chapter.*

1. Which of the following is considered a keyed entry device?
   a. Optical scanner
   b. Mouse
   c. Bar Code reader
   d. Voice recognition

2. The hospital uses six numbers for each patient's medical record. The label on the folder indicates the following number: 31-57-98  6.
   The number 6 is the
   a. redundant number.
   b. check digit.
   c. batch total.
   d. sequencing check.

3. When a laboratory value falls outside a specified range, its outlier detection is a result of a
   a. check digit.
   b. format check.
   c. reasonableness check.
   d. sequence check.

4. Paper forms should include:
   a. instructions/title.
   b. purpose.
   c. user(s).
   d. controls.

5. A data item that contains an eight-digit social security number represents an error detected by
   a. transaction checking.
   b. sequence checking.
   c. reasonableness checking.
   d. format checking.

6. Which of the following would be the most difficult to complete in data entry by health care information staff and which would require the most instructions?
   a. Reimbursement type
   b. Cell type of cancer, based on information in pathology report
   c. Next of kin
   d. Stage of cancer at diagnosis

Questions 7 and 8 present data commonly found in the health care information setting. From the alphabetical list below, choose the letter of the appropriate category each represents. When two possible categories exist, select the "best".

   a. Numeric/integer
   b. Text/character/category
   c. Memo
   d. Date
   e. Time
   f. Logic

7. 250.10, 410.9 [ICD-9-CM code field]

8. Smith [attending physician field]

9. Identify the error in the following coding scheme for race of patient.
   1 = White
   2 = Black
   3 = Asian
   4 = Jewish
   5 = American Indian
   6 = Other

10. The information system shown below was set up for a college's Dental Hygiene Program Clinic in which they wanted to track information about individual patients as well as student activity as it related to treatment of these patients. The following three tables, of many, were incorporated into the database. The relational field that links the VISIT table and the PATIENT table is the

   a. Student number
   b. Patient number
   c. Date of visit
   d. Patient last name

| Patient | Student | Visit |
|---|---|---|
| Patient Number | Student number | Patient Number |
| Patient Last Name | Student Last Name | Date of Visit |
| Patient First Name | Student First Name | Calculus Classification Code |
| Patient Address | Student Address | Gum Disease Code |
| Patient City | Student City | Treatment Code |
| Patient State | Student State | Student Number |
| Patient Zip | Student Zip | |
| Patient Birthdate | Student Telephone Number | |
| | Date of College Admission | |
| | Date of Graduation | |

*Additional review questions can be found on the CD-ROM.*

# Assignments

## 4-1: COMPUTERIZING THE HEALTH INFORMATION FUNCTIONS

### Assignment:

*Prepare a proposal for the purchase of a personal computer for use by the manager of the health information management department in a large physician group practice. Include in the proposal:*

1. The computer specifications: These specifications should be defined so that those not knowledgeable about computers would understand the terminology.
   A. RAM
   B. Hard drive – size
   C. Type of processor
   D. Network connections
   E. MgHz
   F. Additional drives, e.g., CD and speed
2. Types of software – not name brands but functions performed by the software, e.g., word processing, spreadsheet, etc.
3. Justify these purchases by identifying the types of work that can be done more effectively and efficiently on a PC.
4. Illustrate examples of these purchases with ads from store advertisements in print or available from the Internet.
5. Using the examples, prepare a summary sheet with specifications and costs for all of the above items.

## 4-2: PROFESSIONAL PRACTICE EXPERIENCE: PERSONNEL SATISFACTION WITH DATA ENTRY DEVICE

### Assignment:

1. Contact a health care facility that has extensive computerization of its health information systems.
2. Identify and describe the types of automated data input devices currently used (bar code readers, scanning devices, etc.). Describe how they are used.
3. Develop a questionnaire to evaluate the personnel satisfaction with the data entry method currently in use.
4. Administer the questionnaire.
5. Prepare a report showing the results of the survey, analysis of the results and recommendations for improvement.

## 4-3: COMPUTER TOPIC PRESENTATION

## Assignment:

*Select one of the situations below to prepare and deliver a presentation utilizing computer presentation software.*
*The presentation must meet the following criteria:*

- The presentation must contain at least 6 slides – more than 6 may be used.
- Slide 1 will be the title of the presentation, presenter, and audience.
- The remainder of the slides must use at least 5 different slide layouts/formats incorporating a variety of the software's features such as graphics, transitions/animation, different colors, sounds, designs, etc.
- The presentation must fit on removal media, i.e., disk or CD, not a hard drive without the need to condense (pack and go.)
- Text size must be readable by people in the back row of a room.
- Slides must be simple, not containing too many words or ideas.
- Handouts showing six slides to a page should accompany the presentation. If you are using a color printer, you may print the slides in color. If you are using a black and white printer, be sure to have it print in pure black and white.
- References are included in a works sited page. References should be from sources published within the last year. Possible sources of information include vendors. the Internet, recent publications, list-serves, and HIM professionals working in the setting specified.
- Turn in the handout along with the diskette to the instructor after the class presentation.

## Grading:

### Content (35 points possible)

35 = Depth of information appropriate to the topic.

25 = Information somewhat superficial or too detailed.

15 = Little information actually given.

### Presentation (30 points possible)

30 = Clear, easy to follow, did not read all or most of speech. Good eye contact.

20 = Somewhat vague, could not follow at times, or read most of speech. Eye contact poor.

10 = Presentation given, poorly done. No eye contact.

### Presentation Slides (35 points possible)

35 points will be given if the slides and handouts meet all of the requirements above, are neat and professional. 5 points will be deducted from the total points for each of the following errors:

- Slide 1 is not a title slide.
- Less than 5 formats are used — 5 points for each missing layout will be deducted. As an example, if only slides 1, 2, and 3 are different, a total of 15 points will be deducted for slides 4, 5, and 6 that are repeats of other formats.
- No animation is used.

- No transitions are used.
- No sounds are used.
- Typographical/grammar/capitalization errors (instructor subjective judgment on the number of points deducted based on the volume of errors).
- The overall presentation is not professional in appearance (instructor subjective judgment on the number of points deducted based on the overall quality of the slides/handout submitted).

## Topics:

- The current status of voice recognition technology for dictation/transcription systems in health care. Contact software vendors of such systems to determine the state of the art. Check the Internet, recent publications, and/or the HIM-L listserv to obtain recent information.
- Biomedical devices that communicate data directly into patient records. Identify the functions, the data maintained in the record, and the health care setting where these devices are used.
- The current state of the art in computerized data collection and transmission by nurses and other care providers in home health agencies that utilize electronic health records.
- The computer/assistive technology available to assist visually impaired medical transcriptionists and/or other disabled workers.

## 4-4: SELECTION OF DATABASE SOFTWARE

### Assignment:

*In a table format, compare the pros and cons of three "off the shelf" relational database software programs that are available for a personal computer, e.g., for effective use in a health information setting.*

## 4-5: USING DATABASE SOFTWARE IN A MENTAL HEALTH CLINIC

### Assignment:

*Identify and describe those activities in the HIM Department in a mental health clinic that could be done on a personal computer using programs designed with a personal computer relational database software program.*

## 4-6: DEVELOPING A DATABASE FOR EDUCATION/TRAINING INFORMATION

### Assignment:

*Develop a relational database on a personal computer to track education/training information on the employees of a health information department. Include in the data base information on:*

- The health information functions each employee has been trained to do
- The internal inservice programs attended – dates, topic, number of contact hours
- Outside continuing education activities attended – dates, topic, number of contact hours, location, sponsoring association

*Include in the description of the database:*

1. For each field for each employee specify the name, the size, and the types of data.
2. The tables
3. The coding system
4. Validity checks, accuracy and completeness checks used
5. The reports that can be generated from this database
6. Other observations and insights from developing this database

## 4-7: INCIDENT REPORT DATA ENTRY FORM

### Assignment:

*To assist the risk manager, the health information manager developed a personal computer relational database to collect, analyze and report data on incidents. It contains the following six tables:*

1. Identity Table: Provides the code number of the type of person who was injured, e.g., inpatient, visitor, employee, etc.
2. Doctor Table: Doctor number, doctor name, phone and specialty.
3. Location Table: Code number and location (floor) where incident occurred, e.g., First-North, ER, etc.
4. Nature Table: Code number and description of the type of injury, e.g., fracture, broken tooth, etc.
5. Cause Table: Code number and description of the cause of the injuries, e.g., Fall—improper footwear, medication—wrong dosage, etc.
6. Master Table: Lists all codes and other data for each incident as it occurs. The fields in this table are as follows:
   A. Control number
   B. Date of incident
   C. Time of incident
   D. Initials of person who reported incident
   E. Code for identity of person involved in the incident
   F. Record number if person involved was a patient
   G. Age of person involved in incident
   H. Sex of person involved in incident

I. Location of incident
J. Nature of injury
K. Cause of incident
L. Whether or not the physician was notified
M. Whether or not the person was seen by a physician
N. Code number of the physician involved in the case

## Directions:

1. Design an Incident Report to serve as:
   A. Evidence of the incident maintained in the risk manager's files.
   B. The source document for the data entry operator.

   The following should be considered in designing the form:
   - Principles of forms design included in Chapter 4.
   - Inclusion of all codes needed for data entry with the exception of the physician's code numbers. Including the code numbers will speed completion by allowing for checking off the appropriate item and data entry. Because 250 physicians are on staff, their code numbers can be obtained from a separate list and entered into the appropriate part of the form.
   - Length of one or two pages
   - Have spaces for narratives or text entry as needed.
   - Space included to document information for all of the fields listed in the Master Table.

2. Design a computer screen to enter the data from the paper form designed in step 1. While the screen form needs a field to enter each item listed in the Master Table, only a small space is needed to enter the particular code number checked on the form applicable to that patient or visitor who had the injury. The entire list of code numbers does not need to be retyped on the computer screen form. For example, while on the paper form a list needs all nine codes for the Location of Incident field, only two spaces need to be saved on the computer screen to type the information using the keyboard.

3. Explain how properly designed data input paper forms and computer screen forms assist in data quality.

## Coding Scheme:

The coding scheme for the fields are as follows:

### Identity of person

1 = Inpatient

2 = Outpatient

3 = Visitor

4 = Employee

5 = Other

### Sex of person

M = Male

F = Female

O = Other

**Physician code**

(a separate listing of all physicians on staff with a code number next to each physician's name)

**Physician notified**

Y = Yes

N = No

**Person seen by MD**

Y = Yes

N = No

R = Patient refused

**Location of incident**

01 = 1 North

02 = 2 North

03 = 3 North

04 = 4 North

05 = Obstetrics

06 = Nursery

07 = Operating Room

08 = Emergency Room

09 = Other

**Nature of the injury**

01 = Abrasion

02 = Allergic Reaction

03 = Broken tooth

04 = Burn

05 = Comatose

06 = Deceased

07 = Fracture/Dislocation

08 = Infection

09 = Laceration

10 = Other

11 = No apparent injury

**Cause of Incident**

01 = Fall - Improper footwear

02 = Fall - Confused/disoriented

03 = Fall - Fainted

04 = Fall - Lost balance

05 = Fall - No restraints

06 = Fall - Patient sedated

07 = Fall - Senility

08 = Fall - Other

10 = Medication - Administered, with no order

11 = Medication - Administered, after discharge

12 = Medication - Duplicate administration

13 = Medication - Wrong dosage

14 = Medication - Omission

15 = Medication - Wrong medicine

16 = Medication - Wrong site

17 = Medication - Wrong time

18 = Medication - Wrong route

19 = Medication - Other

20 = Equipment - Broken/malfunction

21 = Equipment - Missing

22 = Equipment - Other

30 = Surgical event - Burn

31 = Surgical event - Lost specimen

32 = Surgical event - Missing instrument

33 = Surgical event - Missing needles/sponges

34 = Surgical event - Other

40 = Transfusion - Crossmatch error

41 = Transfusion - Failure to monitor

42 = Transfusion - Wrong patient

43 = Transfusion - Other

50 = Other

*This project is based on an original concept developed by Ardis Alfrey, RHIA, Seattle, WA. Revised by Donna Wilde, MPA, RHIA.*

## 4-8: EVENT AND VALIDATION CHECKS

**Assignment:**

*Using the worksheet below, explain event and validation checks including the use and value of each method.*

### Event and Validation Checks Worksheet

| Event/Validation Check | Description | Use | Value |
|---|---|---|---|

Transaction validation:

_____

Sequence check:

_____

Batch totals:

_____

Audit trails:

_____

Duplicate processing:

_____

Format checks:

_____

Reasonableness checks:

_____

Check digits:

_____

## 4-9: EVALUATION OF FORMS/VIEWS

### Case Study:

A Quality Improvement Team has been formed to evaluate the content of the patient record in preparation for the development of an electronic health record. The team needs to evaluate each form for effectiveness, ease of completion, duplicate data items, and following the principles of effective design.

### Assignment:

1. Using the General Design Principles for forms and views from Chapter 4, design a worksheet to evaluate the paper-based forms that comprise a patient record. The worksheet itself should follow the same general principles.
2. Using the worksheet, evaluate the forms provided to you by the instructor.

## 4-10: FORMS DESIGN

### Assignment:

*The form on the next page is used for routine physician admitting orders for a hospice program.*

1. Review the form and list all errors in forms design.
2. Using word processing software computer program, redesign the form using the principles of forms design discussed in Chapter 4. When used, the form will be maintained in a binder with three holes punched on the left side.

**Morgan Town Hospice**
**4433 Douglas Fir Ave. N.**
**Spruce Mountain, WA 00000**

Admit to Morgan Town  ___ Hospice Inpatient Program  ___ Hospice Home Care Program

___ Both Aspects of Program

Patient Name _____

Primary Site _____  Metastatic Sites _____

    Does patient know diagnosis?  ___ Yes  ___ No
    Has patient had  ___ chemotherapy?  ___ radiation therapy?
    Prognosis for life expectence _____

I.   Immediate Needs:
    ___ pain assessment and management    ___ Nursing assessment
    ___ Nausea and vomiting    ___ Family support and education
    ___ GU care    ___ Nutritional assessment
    ___ Bowel management    ___ Other (Specify) _____
    ___ Oxygen

II.   Patient's current pain management profile _____

    * May adjust present dosage of medication after pain
      assessment and then notify me.    ___ Yes    ___ No

III.   Nausea and vomitting:  ___ Phenergan 25 to 50 mg p.o., suppository or injectable every 4 hour prn
          ___ Torecan 10 mg p.o., suppository or injectable every 6 to 8 hours prn
          ___ Other _____

IV.   GU care:    Foley catheter    ___ Irrigate prn    ___ Other _____

V.   Bowel Management:
    ___ Peri-Colace and Senokot may titrate as needed    ___ Enema prn    ___ Other

VI.   Diet:  ___ As tolerated    ___ Tube feedings    Type of feeding tube _____
                                                                                  Name of feeding _____
                                                                                   Flow rate _____

VII.   Miscellaneous orders: _____

_____

I verify that the above Hospice Skilled services are required. This plan will be periodically reviewed by me, the attending physician, and the services furnished while the patient is under my care.

    Signature of Physician _____  Date _____

Continuing medical care at Morgan Town Hospice inpatient Hospice will be provided by
    ___ Myself    ___ Medical Director

Signature of Physician _____

Copyright © 2001 by W.B. Saunders Company. All rights reserved.

## 4-11: ANNUAL REPORT—WORD PROCESSING

### Directions:

1. Review the following two pages that outline the Health Information Management Department's Annual Report for Hospital Administration and the Board of Trustees.
2. Revise this report on a computer using word processing software. Format the report to be neat and professional in appearance utilizing the following features.
   - Table features must be utilized for items 1-11. Incorporate a variety of word processing features such as different font attributes (bold, italics, underline, etc) to make the report visually attractive
   - Spell out abbreviations when appropriate. Correct all spelling, grammar and capitalization errors
   - Use two decimal places for all numbers. Align the numbers on the decimal point.
   - Use column, row, and borderlines as well as shading for BOTH the row and column headings.

### Grading:

A grade of 100% will be given if the report meets all of the requirements above, is neat, and professional. 5% will be deducted from the score for each of the following errors:

- Table feature is not used
- Two decimal places for numbers are not used
- Numbers are not aligned on the decimal point
- Column, row and border lines for row and column headings are not used
- Shading for BOTH row and column headings are not used
- Typographical/grammar/capitalization errors (instructor subjective judgment on the number of points deducted based on the volume of errors)
- Abbreviations are not spelled out
- A variety of word processing features such as the use of different fonts, bold, italics are not used (but don't make it too "busy")
- The overall report is not professional in appearance (instructor subjective judgment on the number of points deducted based on the overall quality of the report submitted.)

**Teslow**

*Page 1 ANNUAL REPORT Health Info mgt. Dept.*
*2000     Johnstone Memorial Hospital*

## HIGHLIGHTS:

During 2000 we had a record # of discharges. Bills
were prepared in 7.9 days which is a 1.25% improvement over 1999
Several innovative computer systems were created for the financial service department and are discuss under special topics.
See below for departmental statistics.

| HOSPITAL | 1998 | 1999 | 2000 | % Change |
|---|---|---|---|---|
| 1. Units processed Admits + 1/8 output) | 19,494 | 20,042 | 21,955 | +9.5% |
| 2. Paid Sick Leave Hours | 1,244.90 | 983.17 | 1,383.44 | + 41% |
| 3. Overtime Hours | 837.25 | 744.25 | 981.25 | +32% |
| 4 Temporary Labor costs | $15,702 | 0 | 113 | + 100% |
| 5. # FTE's (Totla hours for year ÷ by 2080 hours) | 21.57FTE | 22.99FTE | 23.35 | + 10% |
| 6. Cost to procecess each unit Includes salaries, supplices, repairs, microfilm ect.) | $21.38 | $22.03 | $23.72 | + 7.7% |
| 7. # of requests from Ins. Co and attornies | 5, 149 | 5,577 | 6,860 | + 23% |
| 8 Research and special data Requests from medical Record data base | 38 | 70 | 70 | 0% |
| 9 Discharges including Rehab and Newborn) | 10,949 | 11,539 | 12,445 | + 7.9% |
| 10. processing days (# days from date of discharge to printing the bill) Coding, Abstrac | 11 days | 8 days | 7.9 days | - 1.25% |
| 11. # of lines of dictation typed. Excludes Emergency Room dictation | 742,302 lines | 798,297 Lines | 1,144,980 | + 43% |

Copyright © 2001 by W.B. Saunders Company. All rights reserved.

## SPECIAL PROJECTS

A system for on-line entry of CPT codes for medicare outpatient surgery billing was designed and completed with codes automatically transferred to the bill saving duplicate data entry and time for the business office. A system was developed to track outpatient Medicare surgery reimbursement by each CPT code assigned which then allowed for the creating of a logging system for the Director of Finance to reconcile medicare reimbursement with actual charges.

## ANALYSIS OF STATISTICS FROM PAGE ONE

Item 2. High increase due to several hospitalizaitons

Item 3. Overtime to keep up with 9.5% increase in volume

Item 5. Increase due to volume and also providng better service i.e.;
- A. A clerk position was approved to pull charts on weekends saving time for the nursing service.
- B. Dictation ER load transferred to HIM Dept. Reports are now typed and mailed out to follow-up physicians. This was not done before
- C. Coding ER charts for billing purposes. This had been done in the past by the ER physician, but now many charts are being missed and the coding is done later in medical records.,
- D. CPT coding now required on all outpatient medicare surgery cases.

Item 7. Another year-of increases. This year we have been working with Riverside Copy Service to assist us with this heavy load and maintain costs. Analysis of this project will be done later.

Item 10. We continued to work with the 24 hour-task force. The Statistic of 7.9 days excludes The month of October in calculations because coding and grouper revisions slowed down normal processing time. A recent analysis showed that 61% of non-medicare cases are coded and to the Business Office 2 days after discharge. 92 % of all bills including medicare, are in the bussiness office and ready for transmittal to the various insurance companies 15 days after discharge.

Item 11. Some increase is from volume however, there seems to be more consultations (perhaps an increase in severity of illness and an increase in the length of dictation.

# Review Answers

## PRETEST REVIEW ANSWER KEY

### Directions:

1. Correct your Pretest answers with the answers below by placing a slash through the incorrect question number (Example: 8̸) with a pen or pencil of a contrasting color.
2. Record the correct answer by placing a square around the letter of the correct answer.
3. Record the total correct on the Initial Performance Grid in Section 4 of this review manual.
4. Calculate your performance rate and also record on the grid.
5. Promptly locate the correct answer for each question missed in the chapter of the textbook.
6. Proceed to the chapter review if your performance rate was 80% or higher; otherwise, return to the chapter for further study.

### Answers to Pretest Review:

| | | | | |
|---|---|---|---|---|
| 1. | a | | 6. | b |
| 2. | b | | 7. | a |
| 3. | b | | 8. | a |
| 4. | a | | 9. | a |
| 5. | a | | 10. | b |

## CHAPTER REVIEW ANSWER KEY

### Directions:

1. Correct your answers with the answers below by placing a slash through the incorrect question number (Example: 8̸) with a pen or pencil of a contrasting color.
2. Record the correct answer by placing a square around the letter of the correct answer.
3. Record the total correct on the Initial Performance Grid in Section 4 of this review manual.
4. Calculate your performance rate and also record on the grid.
5. Promptly locate the correct answer for each question missed in the chapter of the textbook.
6. Proceed to the next chapter assigned in your study.

### Answers to Chapter Review:

| | | | | |
|---|---|---|---|---|
| 1. | b | | 7. | b |
| 2. | b | | 8. | b |
| 3. | c | | 9. | Jewish (religion, not race). Would cause the need to classify some patients into two categories. |
| 4. | a | | | |
| 5. | d | | | |
| 6. | d | | 10. | b |

# CHAPTER 5

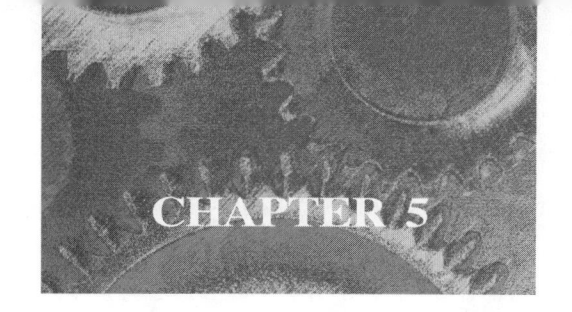

# DATA ACCESS AND RETENTION

## Review

### PRETEST REVIEW

### Directions:

1. Read each question carefully before selecting an answer.
2. Circle the letter of the correct answer.
3. Answer all the questions since there is no penalty for this pretest review.
4. Check your answers with the answer key located at the end of this chapter.

1. The Master Patient Index contains information on inpatients and outpatients.
   a. True
   b. False

2. In a terminal digit filing system, if the number is 64-79-36, the tertiary number is 64.
   a. True
   b. False

3. Scanners are equipment devices basic to optical image processing.
   a. True
   b. False

4. When the destruction of health records policy formation is considered, the governing board should authorize approval of the policy.
   a. True
   b. False

5. To assure that the system will always be available, the optical imaging retrieval workstation should not be capable of running other software.
   a. True
   b. False

6. If a retention schedule is correctly followed, all records can be destroyed after 5 years.
   a. True
   b. False

7. An alphabetic identification system can only be used with an alphabetic filing methodology.
   a. True
   b. False

8. The legality of microfilm is questionable and should be investigated separately in each state.
   a. True
   b. False

9. Records become inactive when the patient expires.
   a. True
   b. False

10. Transfer notices in a permanent filing system have a lower work priority than the retrieval of patient records from the file.
    a. True
    b. False

# CHAPTER REVIEW

## Directions:

1. Read each question carefully before selecting an answer.
2. Circle the letter of the correct answer.
3. Answer all the questions since there is no penalty for this pretest review.
4. Check your answers with the answer key located at the end of this chapter.

| Master Patient Index Screen ||
|---|---|
| Name: Smith, John James | MR#: 12-34-56 |
| DOB: 06-03-1936 | SS#: 294-55-3235 |
| Sex: M | |
| Dates of Admission: | Discharge: |
| 01-10-84 | 01-15-84 |
| 06-05-91 | 06-07-91 |
| 10-20-94 | 10-26-94 |

1. Referring to the information in the box above, what was the date of Mr. Smith's first admission?

2. Referring to the information in the box above, on what day was Mr. Smith discharged on his last admission?

3. Referring to the information in the box above, what is Mr. Smith's first name?

4. Referring to the information in the box above, in what section of the terminal digit filing system would you begin to look for Mr. Smith's record?

5. Referring to the information in the box above, in what month was Mr. Smith born?

6. A jukebox is a component of which system?
    a. optical imaging system
    b. CAR-roll microfilm system
    c. automated record tracking system
    d. computer output microfiche system

7. Which factor would be decreased by using cache memory in an optical imaging system?
    a. exchange time
    b. access time
    c. storage time
    d. video refresh rate

8. A file area that has limited space, low file activity, and one primary file maintenance worker might benefit from choosing which type of filing equipment?
    a. open-shelf filing units
    b. lateral filing cabinets
    c. vertical filing cabinets
    d. motorized revolving units

9. Which of the following is characteristic of an automated record tracking system?
    a. requisition slips are illegible
    b. workload is difficult to prioritize
    c. system is updated in real-time
    d. transfer notices are filed before patient records are retrieved

Copyright © 2001 by W.B. Saunders Company. All rights reserved.

10. Which type of filming method must you choose to maintain the unit record concept and have the microfilm available where the patient is serviced?
    a. roll microfilm
    b. CAR-roll microfilm
    c. jacket microfilm
    d. CAR-jacket microfilm

*Additional review questions can be found on the CD-ROM.*

# Assignments

## 5-1: ST. ANYWHERE COMMUNITY HOSPITAL—DECISION MATRIX ON LONG TERM STORAGE

### Assignment:

*Based on the following scenario, develop a matrix to determine the best alternative for long term storage and retrieval of information at St. Anywhere Community Hospital. Consider the three alternatives of:*

- commercial storage
- microfilm
- optical imaging.

### Scenario:

St. Anywhere Community Hospital has patient records that date back to 1953, when the facility opened. The administration has requested the Director of the Health Information Services to look at the options for storage of these inactive records. The facts about the records and the facility are:

1. All records are paper-based.
2. All records created since 1953 are located at the hospital. Those older than 3 years are located in the basement storage area, with newer records in the main department.
3. Record activity logs show:

   | Age of records: | Requests per week: |
   | --- | --- |
   | 1953 - 1960 | Rare |
   | 1960 - 1970 | 5 |
   | 1970 to present | 50 |

4. Age of the record is not noted on the record folder. It is determined by searching through the folder.
5. The records are clean but many are old and brittle.
6. Laboratory reports are mounted to paper backing sheets with tape on the records located in the basement. Newer records have computer generated full page laboratory reports.
7. The basement storage area contains open shelving units with 28,800 filing inches. The records are packed very tightly on the shelves.
8. The rumor is that Administration is looking for a place to expand the Physical Therapy Department as soon as possible, without any new construction.

## 5-2: ROENTGEN MEMORIAL HOSPITAL—CONSULTANT TO RADIOLOGY SERVICES

### Assignment:

*Develop a consultation report for the Manager of Radiology Services to address the following concerns. Organize the report in the form of a memo with sections labeled "Findings" and "Recommendations":*

### Scenario:

The new Administrator at Roentgen Memorial Hospital asks the Health Information Manager to assist the Manager of Radiology to investigate the findings of a recent satisfaction survey of the medical staff. Referring physicians stated that lost films was their chief concern of service quality. Roentgen Memorial has always prided itself in providing quality radiology services to the community.

The following items were found on the first consulting visit:
1. The X-ray films are filed using a straight numeric methodology, based on a number sequentially assigned within the Radiology Department. A card file that includes the patient's name and x-ray file number is maintained in two large cabinets in the file room. Technicians and clerical staff must reference this file to locate the films. A spot check of the file indicates that duplicate numbers have been assigned.
2. The X-ray jackets are not identified on the outside with the patient record number but the reference copies of reports contained inside the jackets have the patient record number typed on them.
3. The X-ray jackets are manila stock with no color-coding. Outguides and hand-written requisition slips are used in the files.
4. Space is an issue in the department but other storage space is available in a secured, climate-controlled area on the lower level of the hospital.
5. The radiologists use digital dictation to record their report findings and must enter both the patient record number and the x-ray file number as patient identifiers before the system will accept their dictation.
6. The two major problem areas identified by the Radiology Manager are lost x-ray jackets and excessive clerical time required for storage and retrieval of films, including misfile searches.
7. Roentgen Memorial Hospital has a computerized master patient index and patient record tracking software that uses bar code technology. The hospital mainframe vendor has other software available that might be of use.

## 5-3: SMALL BUT BUSY (SBB) CLINIC—MICROFILMING PROPOSAL

### Assignment:

*Write a memo to the administrator to justify the recommendation for the volume microfilming method (microfilming the inactive portions of active records using a microfilm jacket format) to alleviate the record management filing problems for the Small But Busy Clinic. Include in the memo the additional equipment that will be needed to film next year's inactive records at the Small But Busy (SBB) Clinic.*

### Scenario:

The Small But Busy Clinic has a new HIM professional. The clinic has several concerns that affect record management. They are:

1. Increasing Patient Volume: The files of active patients are growing rapidly in size because the staff at SBB are all gerontologists.
2. Filing Space: Shelving space is extremely tight, and the department needs space badly.
3. Revisit Rate: Few files are inactive because the clinic has a very loyal patient population. The physicians and nurses expressed a need to refer to past records to see the evolution of the patients' chronic conditions.
4. Current Procedure for Inactive Records: Records of patients who have not visited SBB for five years are microfilmed on microfilm jackets and stored in the records area.
5. Budget: The administrator mentioned that some funds are available from the operating budget to pay for projects. However, she said that funds are very scarce for the purchase of equipment until the new budget year starts in 6 months. While an optical imaging or computerized alternative may seem like the best solution, the HIM professional realizes that the budget won't allow it now and probably not in the near future.

## 5-4: DOWNTOWN PUBLIC HEALTH CLINIC—TRAINING PROGRAM

### Assignment:

1. Evaluate the scenario below and from the limited information determine the best filing system for the Downtown Public Health Clinic.
2. For the filing system selected in 1, develop a training program for the staff who will be working in the filing and retrieval of patient records.
   A. List the key points to be discussed in the training.
   B. Describe training aids to be used in the training.
   C. Describe the job performance aids that can assist with continuing effective performance after the training is completed.

### Scenario:

The Downtown Public Health Clinic has been open five years. It files its patient records alphabetically by the patient's last name. The staff have spoken of problems locating records.

More than 95% of the clients served by the clinic are on medical assistance. The patient's medical assistance number is their social security number and is already found on the folder cover. The Health Information Manager has suggested that records be filed by this number using a terminal digit methodology. However the nurse manager is concerned that the nine-digit number is too long and will lead to misfiled and lost records.

## 5-5: HILL-BURTON COMMUNITY HOSPITAL—PHARMACY

### Assignment:

*Develop a memo to the Pharmacy Manager for recommendations for the following scenario.*

### Scenario:

The Pharmacy Manager is looking for a more efficient way to store prescription copies of Class II drugs. These prescriptions must be kept permanently by law, but are rarely, if ever, referenced. The prescriptions are on forms that are 4 x 8 inches in size. They are dated with the date of the prescription.

The forms are being stored in date order for two years in a storage area inside the pharmacy and then in a basement storage area. Both areas are now full. The Pharmacy needs the space to create a clean area for preparation of sterile IVs. The Pharmacy Manager knows that the hospital films patient records regularly.

## 5-6: MODERN CLINIC—TRANSCRIPTION

### Assignment:

*Devise the solution to improve the record management functions in the following situation.*

### Scenario:

The Large HMO has just acquired Modern Clinic. The Senior Managers have reported that health information availability is a problem at the Clinic. Investigation reveals:

1. The transcriptionists type reports as dictated, then search for the patient's record to verify patient names, patient numbers and dates of visits from the patient's paper medical record. Once the information is found, it must be added to the report and the report must be re-printed. The records are held in the transcription area until the reports are completed. Transcription is usually two weeks behind.
2. The Clinic has a computerized appointment and billing system on a mainframe computer.
3. The transcriptionists use personal computers and a popular word processing software to create the reports. These computers are networked to each other and not to the mainframe.

## 5-7: MODERN CLINIC—RECORD TRACKING SYSTEM

### Assignment:

*Using the discussion of Chapter 5 obtaining commitment and purchasing agreement for an optical imaging system as a pattern, write the system summary for the automated record tracking system for presentation to the Board of Directors of Modern Clinic.*

### Scenario:

At the Modern Clinic, the manual record tracking system is not meeting the physicians' needs. Because of ineffective systems, clinic staff are circumventing established procedures to get the records to the physicians for patient care.

- When patients go from one clinic area to another, record transfer notices are not used. The transfer notices use special forms and are not easily located in the clinic.
- Requisition forms frequently get lost on their way to the record area.
- The Health Information staff's morale is low because they feel like others are counterproductive to them by relocating records and not telling them.

There is no doubt that an automated record tracking system would help solve some or all of these problems. The clinic's computer vendor has software available to perform all of the functions discussed in the textbook and to provide all the reports that are needed.

## 5-8: ADVANCED TECHNOLOGY HOSPITAL (ATH) ON-LINE OPTICAL IMAGE BASED PATIENT RECORD—COSTS

### Assignment:

*Identify areas where savings can take place within the three major cost categories of 1) equipment, 2) personnel, and 3) overhead.*

### Scenario:

The HIM professional is leading a team at ATH to investigate the possibility of implementing an on-line optical image based patient record. The team has designed a system that combines existing mainframe technology with electronic data interchange (EDI) between systems and computer output to laser disk (COLD).

## 5-9: ADVANCED TECHNOLOGY HOSPITAL (ATH) ON-LINE OPTICAL IMAGE BASED PATIENT RECORD—PERSONNEL

### Assignment:

*Identify the new responsibilities and job titles for the staff when the optical imaging system is implemented. Justify the new positions by including a description of their functions.*

### Scenario:

The current staffing for the Health Information Department of the ATH is as follows(note: 1.0 FTE is 1 full-time equivalent or 40 hours of paid time per week).

### Management

1.0 FTE Health Information Department Director

1.0 FTE Health Information Department Assistant Director

1.0 FTE Record Management Supervisor

### Record Processing

1.0 FTE Record Assembly

2.0 FTE Deficiency Analysis

2.0 FTE Incomplete Record Management Staff

4.0 FTE Permanent Filing Staff

### Coding

1.0 FTE Coding Supervisor

4.0 FTE Coding Specialist

### Release of Information (ROI)

1.0 FTE ROI Supervisor

3.0 FTE ROI Specialist

## 5-10: FILE AREA FLOOR PLANS

### Scenario:

The file room of a health information department in a small hospital occupies 400 square feet of space in a 20' by 20' room. The current floor plan is labeled as Floor Plan #1. The health information professional is planning the budget for the following year and wants to add health record storage space to the room. The existing office furniture must be used but file shelving can be added. Floor plan #2 is the drawing proposed for the following year.

### Assignment:

*Examine both drawings and answer the following questions:*

1. How many filing inches are available in each floor plan?
   Floor Plan #1:
   Floor Plan #2:
2. Which floor plan provides the most quiet work area?
3. List one positive aspect of each floor plan.
   Floor Plan #1:
   Floor Plan #2:
4. List one negative aspect of each floor plan.
   Floor Plan #1:
   Floor Plan #2:

**Floor Plan 1**

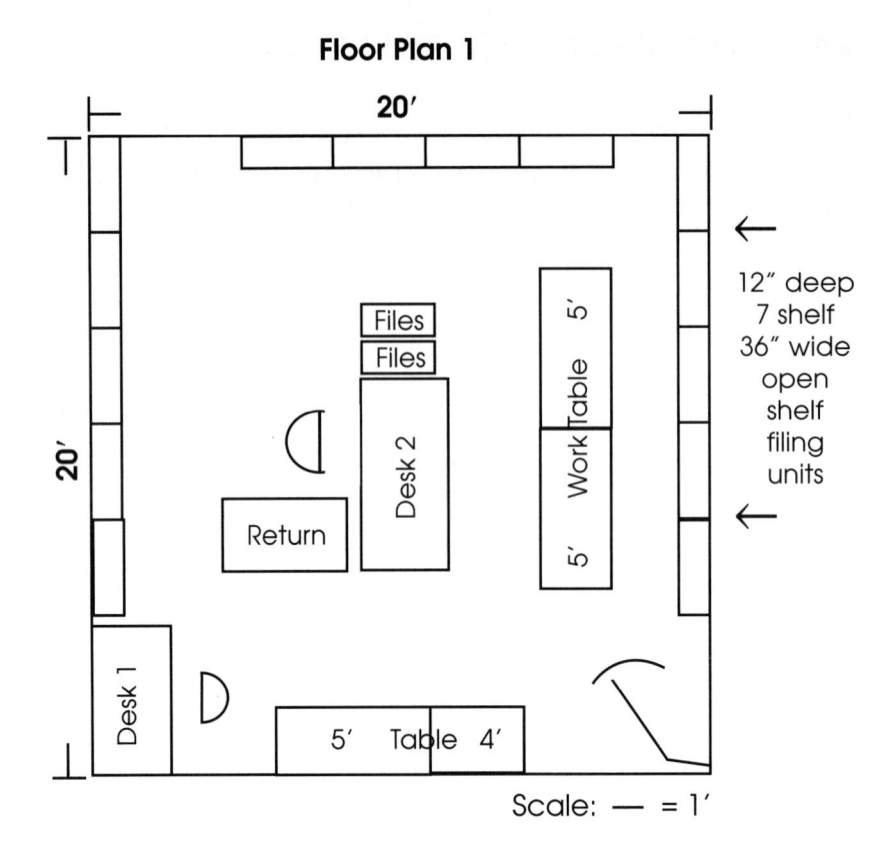

- 20' (width)
- 20' (height)
- Files
- Files
- Desk 2
- Return
- Work Table 5' × 5'
- Desk 1
- 5' Table 4'
- 12" deep 7 shelf 36" wide open shelf filing units

Scale: — = 1'

**Floor Plan 2**

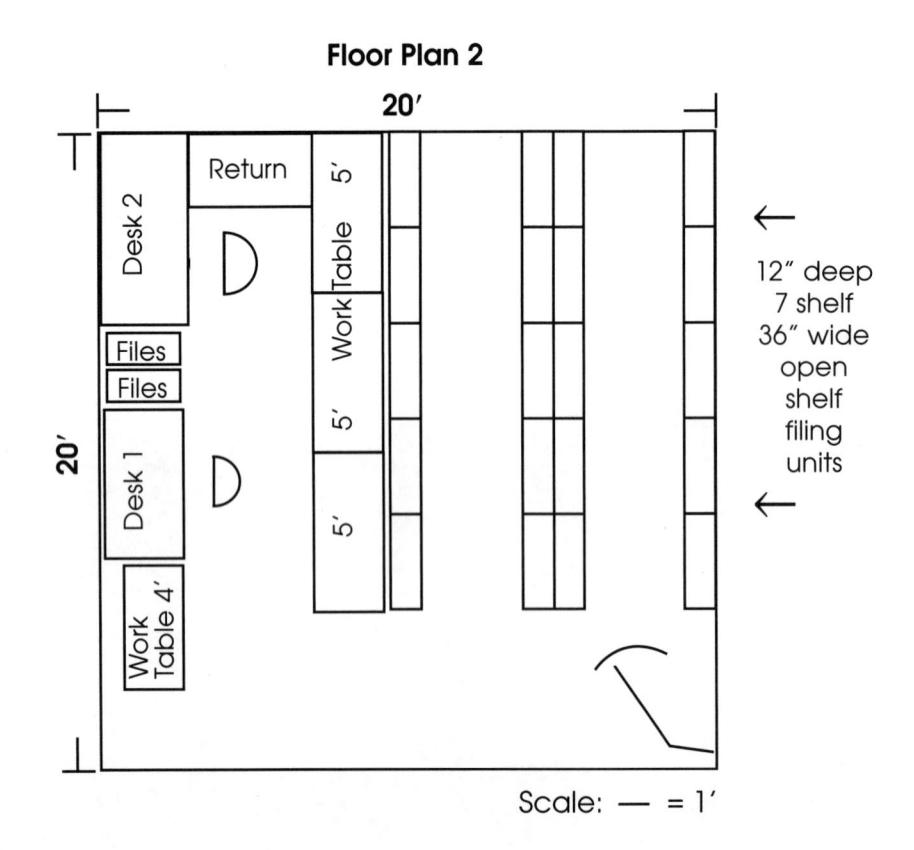

- 20' (width)
- 20' (height)
- Desk 2
- Return
- Work Table 5' × 5'
- Files
- Files
- Desk 1
- Work Table 4'
- 12" deep 7 shelf 36" wide open shelf filing units

Scale: — = 1'

## 5-11: DATA ACCESS AND RETENTION PROGRAM ASSESSMENT

### Assignment:

*Develop a checklist for use in evaluating whether the data access and retention program at a health care facility meets the faculty's current and future needs.*

## 5-12: LONE PINES HOSPITAL IN LITTLETON, WASHINGTON—FILING SPACE

### Scenario:

Lone Pines Hospital in Littleton, Washington is a 35-bed hospital with a small outpatient clinic. The hospital averages 4000 discharges per year and has patient records that average .35 inches each. The retention period in the state of Washington is 10 years.

The Health Information Department, staffed by two FTE, has a space problem. It is very cramped with only 9216 filing inches in 32 open-shelf filing units. It needs 14,000 filing inches.

In the near future, the department will be relocated to a new 256 square (16' x 16') room. XYZ Office Supply, a local shelving vendor, has located a buyer for their existing open-shelf filing units, if they will no longer be needed.

1. Why does the hospital need to have 14,000 filing inches in the new space?
2. If you were the director of the Health Information Department, what type of filing equipment would you purchase for installation at Lone Pines?
3. Develop a report for administration, stating your findings and rationale for your choice of filing equipment.

## 5-13: OLD HEALTH CLINIC—DISPOSITION OF RECORDS ON CLOSURE

### Scenario:

Old Health Clinic is closing at the end of the year. The physician owner, Dr. Miller, is retiring. The building is being demolished and the new owners will use the land for an office building.

### Assignment:

*Create a To Do List of items that need completion for the disposition of patient records with the closure of Old Health Clinic.*

## 5-14: PROFESSIONAL PRACTICE EXPERIENCE—DATA ACCESS AND RETENTION PROGRAMS

### Assignment:

1. Arrange to visit three different types of health care facilities from the following list:
   - Skilled Nursing Facility
   - Physicians' Office (3 or more physicians)
   - Freestanding Ambulatory Surgery Center
   - Hospital
   - Home Health Agency
2. Compare and contrast the data access and retention programs on three different topics discussed in Chapter 5.

## 5-15: QUAD STATE MEDICAL CENTER—RECORD RETENTION

### Scenario:

Quad State Medical Center is a hospital in Oklahoma that also owns specialty physician clinics in Oklahoma, Missouri, Arkansas, and Kansas. All of the clinics are within a 20-mile radius of the hospital. The facility maintains a unit record and the record travels by courier to each location, as needed, for patient appointments/hospitalizations. The physician clinics are licensed to operate in their individual states.

Administration has asked you why patient records need to be maintained for such a long time. They are currently kept for 10 years, even though Oklahoma Department of Health Regulations requires only five years.

### Assignment:

*Write a report to the administrator from the Director of Health Information providing the specifics of why the record retention program currently in place is appropriate.*

## 5-16: PEDIATRICIANS' OFFICE—A NEW ALPHABETICAL FILE

### Scenario:

Three pediatricians are buying the practice of a retiring physician after completing their residency. They have determined that they will use a popular off-the-shelf accounting system to run their practice. It does not support the assignment of a patient record number to patients. Therefore, the physicians feel that they are fairly safe in continuing the use of alphabetic identification and alphabetic filing.

The physicians need assistance in determining how to plan for the expansion of their patient record storage area. They have purchased three additional open-shelf filing units to go with the four units already in place. These units are 8 shelves high and 36" wide.

### Assignment:

*Answer the following questions for this practice:*

1. How many filing inches of space will the new practice have available?
2. How many filing inches will be devoted to each alphabetic section of the files?

## 5-17: TO DECENTRALIZE OR NOT TO DECENTRALIZE, THAT IS THE QUESTION

### Scenario:

Two physicians within a group practice of 10 doctors want to maintain their own patient records in their private office suites. They are willing to consider the pros and cons of the subject.

### Assignment:

*Write a memo to the physicians that outlines the positives and negatives of decentralized filing so that they can make an informed decision.*

## 5-18: THOUGHT QUESTIONS

### Assignment:

1. Define the minimum data elements needed in an automated master patient index.
2. What optional data elements should be considered for inclusion?

## 5-19: LITTLE HOSPITAL—OFF-SITE STORAGE—REQUIREMENTS DOCUMENT FOR A NEW SYSTEM

### Scenario:

Little Hospital has 3 years of inactive patient records that they can no longer store on-site. The hospital would like to use this space for another x-ray examination room within the next 2 months.

Approximately 15,000 records currently occupy 6000 filing inches. These records are retrieved only in 4 percent of the cases each year. The record folders are bar-coded for use with their automated record tracking system. They have no other records stored off-site at the present time. Developing a long-term relationship with an off-site storage company that can take yearly shipments of inactive records is a goal for the Health Information Department.

### Assignment:

*Develop a requirements document for the selection of an off-site storage vendor. Include a section on each of the following:*

Purpose of the request
Definition of terms included in the document
Current status of the paper record storage system, including statistics
Goals for the new system
Terms and conditions that a vendor must meet to gain the business
Response time frame requirements for quotes

## 5-20: METROPOLITAN HOSPITAL—DISASTER RECOVERY

### Scenario:

Metropolitan Hospital suffered a malfunction of the sprinkler system in the incomplete record processing area. There are 864 filing inches of wet records that need to be dried so they can be processed to completion.

The Director of Health Information contacted a restoration specialist by using the ASCR website but the closest one is not in the same city. The truck from a neighboring state will arrive tomorrow morning.

### Assignment:

*Answer the following questions.*

1. What should be done while waiting for the restoration specialists to arrive?
2. What method of restoration will be requested to be used on the records and why?

# Review Answers

## PRETEST REVIEW ANSWER KEY

### Directions:

1. Correct your Pretest answers with the answers below by placing a slash through the incorrect question number (Example: 8) with a pen or pencil of a contrasting color.
2. Record the correct answer by placing a square around the letter of the correct answer.
3. Record the total correct on the Initial Performance Grid in Section 4 of this review manual.
4. Calculate your performance rate and also record on the grid.
5. Promptly locate the correct answer for each question missed in the chapter of the textbook.
6. Proceed to the chapter review if your performance rate was 80% or higher; otherwise, return to the chapter for further study.

### Answers to Pretest Review:

| | | | | |
|---|---|---|---|---|
| 1. | a | 6. | b |
| 2. | a | 7. | a |
| 3. | a | 8. | b |
| 4. | a | 9. | b |
| 5. | b | 10. | b |

## CHAPTER REVIEW ANSWER KEY

### Directions:

1. Correct your answers with the answers below by placing a slash through the incorrect question number (Example: 8) with a pen or pencil of a contrasting color.
2. Record the correct answer by placing a square around the letter of the correct answer.
3. Record the total correct on the Initial Performance Grid in Section 4 of this review manual.
4. Calculate your performance rate and also record on the grid.
5. Promptly locate the correct answer for each question missed in the chapter of the textbook.
6. Proceed to the next chapter assigned in your study.

### Answers to Chapter Review:

| | | | | |
|---|---|---|---|---|
| 1. | 01-10-84 | 6. | a |
| 2. | 26th (10-26-94) | 7. | b |
| 3. | John | 8. | d |
| 4. | 56 | 9. | c |
| 5. | 6th month or June | 10. | c |

Copyright © 2001 by W.B. Saunders Company. All rights reserved.

# CHAPTER 6

# CODING, CLASSIFICATION, AND REIMBURSEMENT SYSTEMS

## Review

### PRETEST REVIEW

**Directions:**

1. *Read each question carefully before selecting an answer.*
2. *Circle the letter of the correct answer.*
3. *Answer all the questions since there is no penalty for this pretest review.*
4. *Check your answers with the answer key located at the end of this chapter.*

1. In the APC classification system, the APC assignment is determined primarily by the ICD-9-CM code for the reason for the visit.
   a. True
   b. False

2. Comorbidities can be found on the history and physical examination record.
   a. True
   b. False

3. DRGs are a prospective case mix payment mechanism for inpatients.
   a. True
   b. False

4. A complication is a condition that is present at admission.
   a. True
   b. False

5. The assignment of a DRG is based on the principal diagnosis and significant operating room procedure, if there was a procedure.
   a. True
   b. False

6. A grouper is used to divide patients into DRGs.
   a. True
   b. False

7. ICD-9-CM is used in hospitals and physician's offices.
   a. True
   b. False

8. HCPCS and CPT are classification systems.
   a. True
   b. False

9. Malpractice insurance expense is taken into consideration in the relative value units of the RBRVS system.
   a. True
   b. False

10. The UHDDS captures data on hospital inpatients.
    a. True
    b. False

# CHAPTER REVIEW

## Directions:

1. *Read each question carefully before selecting an answer.*
2. *Circle the letter of the correct answer.*
3. *Answer all the questions since there is no penalty for this pretest review.*
4. *Check your answers with the answer key located at the end of this chapter.*

1. DSM-IIIR is used primarily in psychiatric facilities.
   a. true
   b. false

2. The system developed to standardize terminology used in the clinical laboratory is
   a. SNOMED
   b. Read codes
   c. ICD-O
   d. LOINC

3. Which of the following is true?
   a. The PRO can change a principal diagnosis but cannot add diagnoses.
   b. The PRO can alter a diagnosis, which cannot be verified by the content of the record.
   c. The PRO can add a diagnosis that may change the DRG.
   d. Both a and c

4. You are a coding supervisor at Rocky Mountain Medical Center and are trying to determine how many inpatient coders you need. You have approximately 1500 discharges including deaths per month and each coder will work 150 hours per month. It has been determined that coders should be allowed 20 minutes to code each record. How many coders do you need?
   a. 2.0
   b. 3.3
   c. 4.2
   d. 4.4

5. All of the following are descriptive of Level I codes in the HCPCS *except*
   a. Level I codes are CPT codes
   b. Level I codes are published every 2 years
   c. Level I codes are numeric
   d. Level I codes are strictly for physician services

6. The number of coders needed to code inpatient cases can be calculated to ensure the workload is handled. The numerator for this equation would be:
   a. total number of records to be coded x number of discharges for the period
   b. number of hours worked per coder for the time period
   c. mean coding time per record x number of discharges and deaths for period
   d. coding time per record x number of discharges for the period

7. Supplemental resources for ICD-9-CM coders in inpatient facilities should include:
   a. encoders
   b. Coding clinic
   c. *CPT Assistant*
   d. both a and b

8. Referring to the information in the box below, what validation item is missing from the PRO DRG validation process?

9. Which diagnosis should be listed first when sequencing codes?
   a. principal diagnosis
   b. primary diagnosis
   c. significant diagnosis
   d. secondary diagnosis

10. All of the following require HCPCS/CPT codes *except:*
    a. patient office visit
    b. hospital ambulatory surgery visit
    c. hospital inpatient visit
    d. hospital outpatient visit

---

**PRO DRG Validation Process**

- Accuracy of coding the principal diagnosis, secondary diagnosis, and procedure codes
- Accuracy of codes on UB-92
- Accuracy of discharge disposition

---

*Additional review questions can be found on the CD-ROM.*

# Assignments

## 6-1: CLASSIFICATION EXERCISE

### Assignment:

*The following assignment is an example of classification of diagnoses and procedures for reasons other than reimbursement, research, and health planning. Completion of this assignment will provide learners with practice in using analytical skills needed to code with the classification systems in use today.*

*Physicians are classified or grouped by their medical specialty. Those specialties are grouped to form clinical departments within the medical staff. The number of departments depends on the number of physicians in the medical staff. To keep track of the number of patients served by each department on the medical staff, patients are often grouped by the medical specialty of their physician who treated them. The specialty is determined by the patient's diagnosis.*

### Directions:

*To classify patients into clinical departments takes several steps.*

1. Using the Definitions of Physician Specialty, determine the specialty that would treat the patient with the listed diagnosis.
2. Using the listing of Clinical Departments for each hospital, specify the clinical department for that patient. If the hospital does not have a clinical department for the specialty, group the patient to a broader category. For example, for a patient whose physician is a cardiovascular surgeon, but the hospital does not have a department of cardiovascular surgery, the patient would be grouped to the surgery department.

### Worksheet

| Diagnosis and Procedures | Physician Specialty | Biggest and Best Anywhere Medical Center | Metropolitan Community Hospital | Little Hospital |
|---|---|---|---|---|
| 1. Diabetes Mellitus Type II Uncontrolled | | | | |
| 2. Congestive Heart Failure | | | | |
| 3. Cholecystitis with Cholecystectomy | | | | |
| 4. Anorexia Nervosa | | | | |
| 5. Bleeding Esophageal Varices | | | | |

Copyright © 2001 by W.B. Saunders Company. All rights reserved.

## Worksheet (continued)

| Diagnosis and Procedures | Physician Specialty | Biggest and Best Anywhere Medical Center | Metropolitan Community Hospital | Little Hospital |
|---|---|---|---|---|
| 6. Cerebrovascular Accident | | | | |
| 7. AIDS | | | | |
| 8. Alzheimer's Disease | | | | |
| 9. Antibiotic resistant tuberculosis | | | | |
| 10. Breast cancer with lumpectomy | | | | |
| 11. Malignant Hypertension | | | | |
| 12. BPH with transurethral resection | | | | |
| 13. Burns, 3rd degree on hands and forearms Full thickness skin grafts to burned areas | | | | |
| 14. Malignant melanoma on shoulders and back | | | | |
| 15. False labor | | | | |
| 16. Fracture left femur, hip replacement surgery | | | | |
| 17. Retinitis Pigmentosa | | | | |
| 18. Myocardial infarction with coronary artery bypass graft | | | | |
| 19. Endometriosis | | | | |
| 20. Acute leukemia | | | | |

## Definition of Physician Specialty

| | |
|---|---|
| Cardiology | Cases having a disease of any part of the cardiovascular system, which includes the heart, conduction systems, arteries, veins, and capillaries. |
| Cardiovascular Surgery | Surgical specialty of the heart and blood vessels |
| Dermatology | Diseases and conditions of the skin, including malignant conditions |
| Endocrinology | Diseases and conditions of the endocrine glands, e.g., thyroid, adrenal glands. |
| Gastroenterology | Diseases and conditions of the digestive system, including the esophagus, stomach, intestines, liver, pancreas, and gallbladder treated by medical and/or endoscopic interventions. |
| Gynecology | Surgical specialty concerned with the study of female reproductive and urinary systems and treatment of the disorders. |
| Infectious Disease | Cases of diseases caused by pathogenic microorganisms, including contagious and noncontagious infections. |
| Internal Medicine/Medicine | Cases of diseases of internal organs, using nonsurgical therapy, except those assigned to a subspecialty. |
| Neonatology/Newborn | Treatment of infants born alive in the hospital. |
| Neurology | Diseases of the central, peripheral, and sympathetic nervous systems, except those that require surgery. |
| Neurosurgery | Surgical specialty concerned with diseases of the central, peripheral, and sympathetic nervous systems. |
| Obstetrics | Surgical specialty concerned with the management of pregnancy, including the prenatal, perinatal, and postnatal stages. |
| Oncology | Cases of patients who have cancer and tumors – both benign and malignant. |
| Ophthalmology | All diseases, injuries, and conditions of the eye and supporting structures regardless of types of therapy, except tumors or sexually transmitted diseases. |
| Orthopedics | Surgical specialty concerned with the musculoskeletal system including prevention of disorders and restoration of function. |
| Otorhinolaryngology | Surgical specialty dealing with the study and treatment of disorders of the ears, nose and throat. |

Copyright © 2001 by W.B. Saunders Company. All rights reserved.

| | |
|---|---|
| Pediatrics | Diseases and conditions of children under 14 years old, including normal growth and development. |
| Plastic and Reconstructive Surgery | Surgical specialty concerned with repair, restoration, and reconstruction of body structures. |
| Psychiatry (Behavioral Health) | Cases of mental illness. |
| Surgery | All cases treated by manual or mechanical means except those that are assigned to a surgical specialty. |
| Urology | Surgical specialty concerned with the study and treatment of the male genitourinary system and female urinary organs. |

## Clinical Departments

| Biggest and Best Anywhere Medical Center | Metropolitan Community Hospital | Little Hospital |
|---|---|---|
| Cardiology | Cardiology | Medicine |
| Cardivascular Sugery | Internal Medicine | Obstetrics-Gynecology |
| Dermatology | Newborn | Newborn |
| Endocrinology | Obstetrics-Gynecology | Surgery |
| Gastroenterology | Ophthalmology | |
| Infectious Diseases | Orthopedics | |
| Internal Medicine | Otorhinolaryngology | |
| Neonatology | Surgery | |
| Neurology | Urology | |
| Neurosurgery | | |
| Obstetrics-Gynecology | | |
| Ophthalmology | | |
| Orthopedics | | |
| Otorhinolaryngology | | |
| Plastic and Reconstructive Surgery | | |
| Proctology | | |
| Psychiatry | | |
| Surgery | | |
| Urology | | |

## 6-2: TRAINING CODERS

### Case Study:

Coders are in short supply in the hospital's geographic area. The local community college has a medical assistant program where the students learn medical terminology, anatomy, and physiology. These medical assistant graduates have trouble finding jobs in their field and are applying for the hospital coding positions.

### Assignment:

*Given these applicants, background, design a training program to prepare them for hospital inpatient and outpatient coding. The program should include initial training as well as continuing education. For each step in the training program, specify the content, the methods, length of time, and the performance level that must be achieved by the trainee to move to the next step.*

## 6-3: CODING POLICIES AND ETHICS

### Assignment:

*Develop a coding policy for a physician's office of seven family practitioners and two obstetricians that addresses the issues listed below. The Coding Policies should also reflect an understanding and compliance with The Standards of Ethical Coding found in Chapter 6 of the book.*

### Issues to be Addressed by Coding Policies

- Directions for reviewing the record to assure the codes are supported by the documentation in the record
- Instructions for coding a record with conflicting documentation
- List of terms and definitions that need to be used in assigning and sequencing codes (such as applicable data sets)
- Instructions for updating coding books (specify the time of year when each classification system is updated)
- Reference materials

## 6-4: PROFESSIONAL PRACTICE EXPERIENCE: ASSESSING THE QUALITY OF CODED DATA

### Assignment:

*The quality of coded data is extremely important to a health care organization. Develop a plan to evaluate the quality of coded data. Include in the plan:*

>the process being evaluated
>
>the positions involved in the evaluation
>
>the position doing the evaluation
>
>method of evaluation
>
>the frequency of the reviews (monthly, quarterly)
>
>the volume of records reviewed.

## 6-5: CONSULTING

### Case Study:

University Medical Associates is an organization of 125 physicians who are on the faculty of the University Medical Center. Besides their teaching responsibilities, they practice at the University Hospital and Clinics. There are 25 different outpatient specialty clinics. The clinics provide service to approximately 80 patients a day.

The Compliance Coordinator for University Medical Associates is responsible for the quality of outpatient coding and improving the physicians' documentation practices in the clinic setting. The Compliance Coordinator is an RHIA with a CCS-P. On visits to the clinic and in reviewing the records, she has noticed the following patterns.

- Denials of payment are only investigated when a patient calls to request resubmission of a claim.
- A significant portion of the clinic's patients are Medicaid recipients.
- CPT codes are assigned based on the physician's check-off on the superbill. Physicians check all procedures done. So multiple CPT codes are submitted when only a few are needed.
- Physician documentation in the clinic records does not reflect the examinations performed, the findings made, and the recommendations for follow-up. Typical notes are: "Patient here for renewal of prescription." "Mrs. X doing fine, to come back in two weeks."

### Assignment:

*Develop a report which advises the clinic physicians and billers on more successful methods of documentation and coding. Be sure the report addresses the situations described above.*

## 6-6: HIRING A CODER

### Scenario:

Three people applied for the coding position in the Health Information Management Department in Central City Hospital. This position is responsible for coding Medicare patients' diagnoses and procedures with the use of an encoder in the automated book format.

The three applicants are:
- an RHIA who has experience in long-term care
- CCS who has worked in a family practice physician's office
- a graduate of a one year Coding Certificate Program which is part of a well respected HIM program. She works as a Medicare Biller in a neighboring hospital.

All three applicants were given a coding test. The coding test consisted of coding five real medical records that happened to be available on the day of the applicants' interview. To be fair, applicants were not allowed to use their own coding books but had to use those owned by the hospital.

All applicants did poorly on the test. The Hospital Biller scored the highest.

### Assignment:

1. Which applicant should be hired? Why? Justify your selection.
2. Identify any problems with the hiring process. Why did the applicants do poorly on the coding test? How should the testing situation be changed to be sure the person hired is qualified for the job?

# Review Answers

## PRETEST REVIEW ANSWER KEY

### Directions:

1. Correct your Pretest answers with the answers below by placing a slash through the incorrect question number (Example: 8) with a pen or pencil of a contrasting color.
2. Record the correct answer by placing a square around the letter of the correct answer.
3. Record the total correct on the Initial Performance Grid in Section 4 of this review manual.
4. Calculate your performance rate and also record on the grid.
5. Promptly locate the correct answer for each question missed in the chapter of the textbook.
6. Proceed to the chapter review if your performance rate was 80% or higher; otherwise, return to the chapter for further study.

### Answers to Pretest Review:

| | | | | |
|---|---|---|---|---|
| 1. | b | | 6. | b |
| 2. | a | | 7. | a |
| 3. | a | | 8. | a |
| 4. | b | | 9. | a |
| 5. | b | | 10. | a |

## CHAPTER REVIEW ANSWER KEY

### Directions:

1. Correct your answers with the answers below by placing a slash through the incorrect question number (Example: 8) with a pen or pencil of a contrasting color.
2. Record the correct answer by placing a square around the letter of the correct answer.
3. Record the total correct on the Initial Performance Grid in Section 4 of this review manual.
4. Calculate your performance rate and also record on the grid.
5. Promptly locate the correct answer for each question missed in the chapter of the textbook.
6. Proceed to the next chapter assigned in your study.

### Answers to Chapter Review:

| | | | | |
|---|---|---|---|---|
| 1. | b | | 6. | d |
| 2. | d | | 7. | d |
| 3. | c | | 8. | accuracy of sequencing |
| 4. | b (1500 x .33)/150 | | 9. | a |
| 5. | b | | 10. | c |

Copyright © 2001 by W.B. Saunders Company. All rights reserved.

# CHAPTER 7

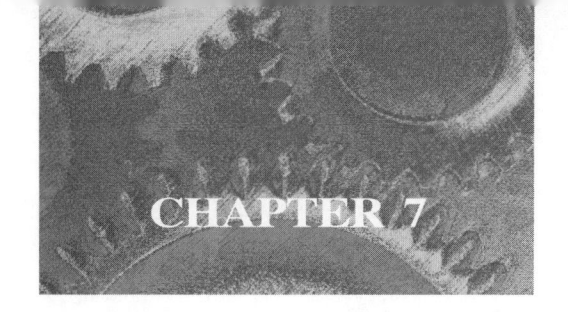

# REGISTRIES

## Review

### PRETEST REVIEW

**Directions:**

1. *Read each question carefully before selecting an answer.*
2. *Circle the letter of the correct answer.*
3. *Answer all the questions since there is no penalty for this pretest review.*
4. *Check your answers with the answer key located at the end of this chapter.*

1. Trauma registries may be hospital or population based.
   a. True
   b. False

2. A case-finding source for a hospital cancer registry includes pathology reports, for example, bone marrow, hematology, and cytology reports.
   a. True
   b. False

3. ICD-O-2 permits coding of neoplastic tissue grades.
   a. True
   b. False

4. A cancer request log should contain the purpose or use of data from each individual requesting data.
   a. True
   b. False

5. A cancer request log should contain the authorization for release of data.
   a. True
   b. False

6. The categories of cancer registries are generally defined as hospital or population-based.
   a. True
   b. False

7. The American College of Surgeons' approved hospital cancer programs are limited to single facility, acute care hospital programs.
   a. True
   b. False

8. The American College of Surgeons requires the cancer committee of a hospital-based cancer registry to meet at least twice a year.
   a. True
   b. False

9. The purpose of a birth defects registry is determined by the type of case ascertainment system it operates.
   a. True
   b. False

10. The Injury Severity Scale is required of trauma registries by the American College of Surgeons.
    a. True
    b. False

# CHAPTER REVIEW

## Directions:

1. *Read each question carefully before selecting an answer.*
2. *Circle the letter of the correct answer.*
3. *Answer all the questions since there is no penalty for this pretest review.*
4. *Check your answers with the answer key located at the end of this chapter.*

1. An annual report is required of cancer registry programs approved by the ACS.
   a. True
   b. False

2. A case-finding source for a hospital cancer registry includes the disease index.
   a. True
   b. False

### Accession Register

| Acc. # | Patient's Name | Primary Site | Site # | Date of Diagnosis |
|---|---|---|---|---|
| 94-0001/00 | Raggedy, A. | Liver | C22 | 01/02/94 |
| 94-0002/02 | Possum, M. | Colon | C18 | 01/03/94 |
| 93-0345/02 | Cake, P. | Lung | C34 | 01/03/94 |
| 94-0004/01 | Doe, John | Prostate | C61 | 01/04/94 |
| 94-0004/02 | Doe, John | Colon | C18 | 01/04/94 |
| 94-0006/00 | Lincoln, M. | Breast | C50 | 01/04/94 |

3. Referring to the data in the table above, A, Raggedy's tumor was not malignant as noted by the accession number.
   a. True
   b. False

4. Referring to the data in the table above, P. Cake was first diagnosed with cancer at this hospital in 1993.
   a. True
   b. False

5. Referring to the data in the table above, there are six different patients—one female and five males.
   a. True
   b. False

6. A cancer registry log should contain the final disposition of the data requested.
   a. True
   b. False

7. The primary goal of hospital-based cancer registries is to:
   a. improve the care of the patient with cancer
   b. monitor local cancer incidence and trends
   c. conduct basic cancer research
   d. assess hospital costs associated with cancer patients

8. How many patient care evaluation studies are required annually by the American College of Surgeons?
   a. one short-term (process)
   b. one long-term (outcome)
   c. one short-term and one long-term
   d. either a short-term or a long-term

9. AIDS cases are identified for inclusion in the registry database using the same case-finding sources used by cancer registries, for example, pathology reports for cancer and oncology patients.
   a. true
   b. false

10. ICD-O-2 permits coding of neoplastic morphology.
    a. True
    b. False

*Additional review questions can be found on the CD-ROM.*

# Assignments

## 7-1: THOUGHT QUESTIONS

### Assignment:

*Answer the following questions.*

1. Define the goals and objectives of patient follow-up in a cancer registry.
2. The integration of computers in cancer registry activities is common. Describe the features of a cancer registry computer system and its advantages.
3. Describe at least four uses of cancer registry data.
4. Similar to Health Information Management, cancer registry professionals are often described as technical (cancer registry technicians) or administrative (cancer program managers). Describe three activities usually associated with each.
5. Select one of the following registries and describe its purpose and common uses of data as described in Chapter 7:
   - birth defects
   - diabetes mellitus
   - trauma
6. List six data variables collected by a trauma registry that are different than those usually included in cancer registry data bases.

## 7-2: CANCER REGISTRY ACCESSION LIST

## Assignment:

*Prepare an accession register by assigning numbers and listing patients described below in the correct order.*

### Patients

Brown, B., localized colon cancer, diagnosed 2/12/00

Jones, T., localized prostate cancer and in situ bladder cancer diagnosed 1/15/00

Smith, J., breast cancer with regional spread, diagnosed 6/25/00

Blue, A., localized lung cancer, diagnosed 4/10/00

Black, S., lung cancer, stage unknown, diagnosed 1/12/00

Red, T., in situ breast cancer, diagnosed 5/1/00

Green, J., stomach cancer with distant metastases, diagnosed 9/1/00

Yellow, C., localized liver cancer, diagnosed 9/2/00

Orange, D., localized prostate cancer, diagnosed 8/25/00

Pink, P., localized breast cancer, diagnosed 8/15/00

Purple, W., colon cancer with regional metastases, diagnosed 7/4/00

White, B., localized brain cancer, diagnosed 3/30/00

Lavender, L., history of breast cancer, new localized colon cancer diagnosed 6/12/00

Blue, A., prostate cancer with bone metastases, diagnosed 10/10/00

Jones, T., leukemia diagnosed 10/30/00

White, M., lung cancer with brain metastases, diagnosed 11/13/00

Blue, A., localized bladder cancer, diagnosed 10/11/00

Green, B., pancreas cancer, stage unknown, diagnosed 12/30/00

Gray, C., colon cancer with regional spread, diagnosed 12/3/00

Tan, B., in situ cervical cancer, diagnosed 11/28/00

Doe, J., lung cancer with brain metastases, diagnosed 5/26/00

Smith, G., localized prostate cancer, diagnosed 12/15/00

Doe, J., lymphoma, diagnosed 5/24/00

Grey, S., cancer, primary unknown, diagnosed 4/3/00

## 7-2: CANCER REGISTRY ACCESSION LIST

### Worksheet
### Cancer Registry
### 2000 Accession List

| Accession Number | Patient Name | Primary Site | Date Of Diagnosis |
|---|---|---|---|
|  |  |  |  |
|  |  |  |  |
|  |  |  |  |
|  |  |  |  |
|  |  |  |  |
|  |  |  |  |
|  |  |  |  |
|  |  |  |  |
|  |  |  |  |
|  |  |  |  |
|  |  |  |  |
|  |  |  |  |
|  |  |  |  |
|  |  |  |  |
|  |  |  |  |
|  |  |  |  |
|  |  |  |  |
|  |  |  |  |
|  |  |  |  |
|  |  |  |  |
|  |  |  |  |

Copyright © 2001 by W.B. Saunders Company. All rights reserved.

## 7-3: PRIMARY SITE TABLE

### Assignment:

*Using the patients listed in Assignment 7-2 and the worksheet below, prepare a primary site table for an annual report.*

**Worksheet**
**2000 Primary Site Table**

| Site | Total | % | Stage ||||| 
|---|---|---|---|---|---|---|---|
| | | | IS | LOC | REG | DIST | UNK |
| | | | | | | | |
| | | | | | | | |
| | | | | | | | |
| | | | | | | | |
| | | | | | | | |
| | | | | | | | |
| | | | | | | | |
| | | | | | | | |
| | | | | | | | |
| | | | | | | | |
| | | | | | | | |
| | | | | | | | |
| Total | | | | | | | |

Key: IS = In situ; LOC = Localized; REG = Regional; DIST = Distant; UNK = Unknown

## 7-4: PROPOSAL FOR A HOSPITAL CANCER PROGRAM

## Assignment:

*Prepare a proposal to Administration for the implementation of a hospital cancer program to include:*
- A. Benefits
- B. Basic components
- C. Staffing
- D. Space/equipment
- E. Projected costs

# Review Answers

## PRETEST REVIEW ANSWER KEY

### Directions:

1. Correct your Pretest answers with the answers below by placing a slash through the incorrect question number (Example: 8) with a pen or pencil of a contrasting color.
2. Record the correct answer by placing a square around the letter of the correct answer.
3. Record the total correct on the Initial Performance Grid in Section 4 of this review manual.
4. Calculate your performance rate and also record on the grid.
5. Promptly locate the correct answer for each question missed in the chapter of the textbook.
6. Proceed to the chapter review if your performance rate was 80% or higher; otherwise, return to the chapter for further study.

### Answers to Pretest Review:

| | | | | |
|---|---|---|---|---|
| 1. | a | 6. | a |
| 2. | a | 7. | b |
| 3. | a | 8. | b |
| 4. | a | 9. | a |
| 5. | b | 10. | b |

## CHAPTER REVIEW ANSWER KEY

### Directions:

1. Correct your answers with the answers below by placing a slash through the incorrect question number (Example: 8) with a pen or pencil of a contrasting color.
2. Record the correct answer by placing a square around the letter of the correct answer.
3. Record the total correct on the Initial Performance Grid in Section 4 of this review manual.
4. Calculate your performance rate and also record on the grid.
5. Promptly locate the correct answer for each question missed in the chapter of the textbook.
6. Proceed to the next chapter assigned in your study.

### Answers to Chapter Review:

| | | | | |
|---|---|---|---|---|
| 1. | a | 6. | b |
| 2. | a | 7. | a |
| 3. | b | 8. | c |
| 4. | a | 9. | a |
| 5. | b | 10. | a |

# CHAPTER 8

# STATISTICS

## Review

### PRETEST REVIEW

### Directions:

1. *Read each question carefully before selecting an answer.*
2. *Circle the letter of the correct answer.*
3. *Answer all the questions since there is no penalty for this pretest review.*
4. *Check your answers with the answer key located at the end of this chapter.*

1. A graph that includes continuous interval categories on the X-axis is a histogram.
   a. True
   b. False

2. Ranked data are discrete data.
   a. True
   b. False

3. A bar graph displays the frequency of variables on the Y-axis.
   a. True
   b. False

4. The Y-axis is the horizontal axis.
   a. True
   b. False

5. A frequency distribution can be used to group ordinal data and their total number of observations.
   a. True
   b. False

6. The NCHS collects data on births, deaths, and fetal deaths.
   a. True
   b. False

7. The numerical expression 10:1 is called a proportion.
   a. True
   b. False

8. 1 in 100,000 is an expression of a rate.
   a. True
   b. False

9. A death occurring within 48 hours after surgery is calculated in the postoperative death rate.
   a. True
   b. False

10. The null hypothesis is stated as if no differences between two groups exist.
    a. True
    b. False

Copyright © 2001 by W.B. Saunders Company. All rights reserved.   131

## CHAPTER REVIEW

### Directions:

1. Read each question carefully before selecting an answer.
2. Circle the letter of the correct answer.
3. Answer all the questions since there is no penalty for this pretest review.
4. Check your answers with the answer key located at the end of this chapter.

1. The anesthesia death rate can be referred to as a cause-specific death rate.
   a. True
   b. False

2. The denominator for the postoperative death rate is the total number of operative procedures for the period.
   a. True
   b. False

### Rocky Mountain Hospital Monthly Report

| July 1995 | Hospital Statistics |
|---|---|
| Discharges (including deaths) | 1099 |
| Total deaths: | 55 |
| Inpatient (incl. 2 coroner's cases) | 51 |
| Outpatient | 4 |
| Total autopsies | 11 |
| Inpatient | 10 |
| Outpatient | 1 |

3. Referring to the data in the report below, the net autopsy rate is:
   a. 19.0%
   b. 20.0%
   c. 20.4%
   d. 22.5%

4. Nosocomial infections are those infections:
   a. occurring 72 hours after admission
   b. occurring less than 72 hours before admission
   c. occurring after surgery
   d. both a and c

5. If a p-value of .001 was obtained, the researcher would most likely:
   a. accept the null hypothesis
   b. reject the null hypothesis
   c. reject the alternative hypothesis
   d. none of the above

6. If a researcher accepts the null hypothesis when it is false, he has committed a type II error.
   a. True
   b. False

7. Which is true regarding comorbidities?
   a. they are a pre-existing condition
   b. they generally increase the length of stay
   c. they affect mortality and morbidity rates
   d. all of the above

8. What was the median length of stay for these psychiatric patients: 4, 11, 2, 1, 8, 22, 7.
   a. 4 days
   b. 7 days
   c. 8 days
   d. none of the above

9. Referring to question #8, the range for these patients' length of stay was:
   a. 7
   b. 13
   c. 21
   d. none of the above

10. Referring to the table below, what was the mean LOS for patients having community-acquired viral pneumonia?

### Length of Stay (LOS)
### Patients with Viral Pneumonia

| Community Acquired | | Nosocomial | |
| MR# | LOS | MR# | LOS |
| --- | --- | --- | --- |
| 207658 | 20 | 123579 | 15 |
| 214592 | 10 | 275816 | 22 |
| 221459 | 7 | 254137 | 18 |
| 158645 | 14 | 321096 | 10 |
| 129876 | 8 | 153992 | 8 |
| Mean = | _____ | Mean = | _____ |
| Median = | _____ | Median = | _____ |

*Additional review questions can be found on the CD-ROM.*

# Assignments

### 8-1: MEASURES OF CENTRAL TENDENCY PROBLEMS

## Assignment:

1. Briefly define:
   A. Mean
   B. Median
   C. Mode
2. For the following groups of numbers compute the mean, median, and mode.

   | A. | B. | C. |
   |---|---|---|
   | 4 | 16 | 5 |
   | 24 | 8 | 6 |
   | 92 | 16 | 7 |
   | 82 | 12 | 8 |
   | 24 | 12 | 8 |
   | 32 | 7 | 8 |
   | 24 | | |

3. Rank the following set of numbers from the highest to the lowest.
   40, 30, 20, 20, 20, 40, 60
4. If 49,487 people died from lung cancer out of 1,478,000 deaths during a calendar year, what is the rate of deaths due to lung cancer per 100 deaths?
5. Out of 26,492 births, 869 males and 642 females were born with birth defects what would be the ratio of males to females born with birth defects?

   What is the rate of babies born with birth defects?

## 8-2: MEASURES OF CENTRAL TENDENCY IN HIM

### Assignment:

*Using the data for Anywhere Health Care Facility, compute the measures of central tendency showing the formula, your work, and answer.*

**Retained Documents/Boxes per Department**
**Anywhere Health Care Facility**

| Department | No. of Documents | No. of Boxes |
| --- | --- | --- |
| Medical Records | 150,000 | 200 |
| Personnel | 10,000 | 13 |
| Radiology | 5,000 | 7 |
| Finance | 3,000 | 4 |
| Clinical Laboratory | 6,000 | 8 |
| Total | 174,000 | 232 |

1. Mean number of documents
2. Mean number of boxes
3. Median number of documents
4. Median number of boxes
5. Standard deviation for the number of documents
6. Standard deviation for the number of boxes

## 8-3: LENGTH OF STAY STATISTICS

**A. Compute the length of stay for this group of acute care patients.**

1. What is the LOS for each patient?

   | Admitted | Discharged | LOS |
   |---|---|---|
   | 10-1-00 | 11-1-00 | _____ |
   | 9-3-00 | 9-29-00 | _____ |
   | 1-4-00 | 2-7-00 | _____ |
   | 3-10-00 | 3-15-00 | _____ |
   | 4-7-00 | 4-14-00 | _____ |

2. What are the total discharge days?
3. What is the average LOS for these five patients?
4. What is the median LOS?

**B. Compute the LOS for this group of long-term care facility patients.**

1. What is the LOS for each patient?

   | Admitted | Discharged | LOS |
   |---|---|---|
   | 9-1-99 | 7-3-00 | _____ |
   | 1-3-00 | 4-15-00 | _____ |
   | 2-14-97 | 5-30-00 | _____ |
   | 7-15-98 | 9-2-00 | _____ |

2. What are the total discharge days?
3. What is the average LOS for these four patients?
4. What is the median LOS?

## C. LOS for patients discharged on 6-23-00.

1. What is the length of stay for each patient discharged on 6-23-00?

   | Patient | Admitted | LOS |
   |---------|----------|-----|
   | #1 | 6-1-00 | _____ |
   | #2 | 6-8-00 | _____ |
   | #3 | 6-10-00 | _____ |
   | #4 | 6-14-00 | _____ |
   | #5 | 6-15-00 | _____ |
   | #6 | 6-15-00 | _____ |
   | #7 | 6-16-00 | _____ |
   | #8 | 6-17-00 | _____ |
   | #9 | 6-18-00 | _____ |
   | #10 | 6-19-00 | _____ |
   | #11 | 6-19-00 | _____ |
   | #12 | 6-19-00 | _____ |
   | #13 | 6-19-00 | _____ |
   | #14 | 6-19-00 | _____ |
   | #15 | 6-19-00 | _____ |
   | #16 | 6-19-00 | _____ |
   | #17 | 6-19-00 | _____ |
   | #18 | 6-20-00 | _____ |
   | #19 | 6-19-00 | _____ |
   | #20 | 6-20-00 | _____ |
   | #21 | 6-20-00 | _____ |
   | #22 | 6-20-00 | _____ |
   | #23 | 6-20-00 | _____ |
   | #24 | 6-20-00 | _____ |
   | #25 | 6-21-00 | _____ |
   | #26 | 6-22-00 | _____ |
   | #27 | 6-21-00 | _____ |

2. What is the total LOS for all patients in the above group?  _____
3. What is the ALOS for the above patients?  _____

**D. Compute the average length of stay (ALOS) for these clinical services for August, 2000.**

1. What is the ALOS for patients discharged from each clinical service?

   | Service  | # Pts. Disch | Disch Days | Census Days | ALOS |
   |----------|--------------|------------|-------------|------|
   | Medicine | 307          | 2472       | 2512        | ____ |
   | Surgery  | 462          | 2368       | 2412        | ____ |
   | OB       | 147          | 325        | 347         | ____ |
   | NB       | 148          | 307        | 315         | ____ |

2. What is the ALOS for all four nursing units?

# E. Length of stay by clinical service:

1. What is the LOS for each patient?

| Name | Age | Service | Adm | Disch | LOS |
|---|---|---|---|---|---|
| Johnson | 42 | MED | 6-1 | 6-5 | _____ |
| Pauls | NB | NB | 5-27 | 6-6 | _____ |
| Peabody | 31 | Surg | 4-22 | 6-7 | _____ |
| Patton | NB | NB | 5-28 | 6-5 | _____ |
| Lundstrom | 11 | Surg | 5-26 | 6-8 | _____ |
| Lyons | NB | NB | 5-26 | 6-7 | _____ |
| Maag | 42 | Med | 5-21 | 6-6 | _____ |
| Luther | 54 | OB | 5-21 | 6-6 | _____ |
| Lowe | 63 | Med | 5-20 | 6-5 | _____ |
| Gray | 67 | Surg | 5-19 | 6-7 | _____ |
| Grant | 82 | Med | 6-3 | 6-8 | _____ |
| Green | 97 | Surg | 6-1 | 6-9 | _____ |
| Epp | 80 | Med | 5-19 | 6-7 | _____ |
| Enterkin | 27 | Surg | 5-19 | 6-5 | _____ |
| England | 31 | Med | 5-21 | 6-6 | _____ |
| Cora | 40 | Surg | 5-19 | 6-7 | _____ |
| Cox | 32 | Surg | 5-21 | 6-9 | _____ |
| Craig | 31 | Med | 5-22 | 6-3 | _____ |
| Cotter | 61 | OB | 5-27 | 6-4 | _____ |
| Cornish | 59 | OB | 5-22 | 6-5 | _____ |
| Anderson | 57 | Med | 5-19 | 6-6 | _____ |
| Amos | 48 | Surg | 5-22 | 6-8 | _____ |
| Huber | 34 | Surg | 6-2 | 6-5 | _____ |
| Howes | 37 | Med | 6-3 | 6-8 | _____ |
| Nightengale | 52 | Med | 6-4 | 6-9 | _____ |

2. What is the total LOS for all patients?  _____
3. What is the total number of discharges?  _____
4. What is the total LOS and ALOS by clinical department?  _____

|  | Total | ALOS |
|---|---|---|
| Medicine | _____ | _____ |
| Surgery | _____ | _____ |
| OB | _____ | _____ |
| NB | _____ | _____ |

5. What is the average age of the above patients (excluding NB)? _____

**F. Compute the total number of patients, total LOS and ALOS for each service.**

| Medicine | | Surgery | | OB | | NB | | Total | |
|---|---|---|---|---|---|---|---|---|---|
| # Pts. | Days | # Pts. | Days | # Pts. | Days | # Pts. | Days | # Pts. | Days |
| 18 | 94 | 15 | 119 | 5 | 23 | 4 | 17 | ___ | ___ |
| 4 | 36 | 11 | 61 | 8 | 32 | 7 | 29 | ___ | ___ |
| 8 | 37 | 4 | 61 | 4 | 19 | 4 | 26 | ___ | ___ |
| 6 | 62 | 14 | 140 | 9 | 42 | 8 | 36 | ___ | ___ |
| 8 | 61 | 14 | 108 | 13 | 57 | 9 | 41 | ___ | ___ |
| 13 | 95 | 12 | 72 | 3 | 11 | 2 | 9 | ___ | ___ |
| 12 | 60 | 18 | 115 | 9 | 32 | 6 | 22 | ___ | ___ |
| 6 | 33 | 19 | 145 | 11 | 44 | 8 | 30 | ___ | ___ |
| 6 | 36 | 11 | 65 | 4 | 17 | 3 | 14 | ___ | ___ |
| 4 | 23 | 19 | 216 | 9 | 36 | 7 | 32 | ___ | ___ |
| 3 | 8 | 18 | 130 | 2 | 6 | 2 | 6 | ___ | ___ |
| 9 | 112 | 20 | 217 | 7 | 31 | 7 | 27 | ___ | ___ |
| 10 | 101 | 20 | 144 | 7 | 34 | 7 | 33 | ___ | ___ |
| 8 | 75 | 26 | 262 | 9 | 31 | 4 | 16 | ___ | ___ |
| 5 | 66 | 28 | 377 | 9 | 35 | 7 | 31 | ___ | ___ |
| 7 | 84 | 14 | 96 | 10 | 36 | 6 | 25 | ___ | ___ |
| 7 | 71 | 12 | 114 | 5 | 14 | 3 | 11 | ___ | ___ |
| 3 | 35 | 23 | 172 | 2 | 9 | 3 | 17 | ___ | ___ |
| 8 | 62 | 28 | 236 | 10 | 55 | 5 | 27 | ___ | ___ |
| 12 | 82 | 22 | 117 | 10 | 60 | 9 | 54 | ___ | ___ |
| 11 | 86 | 24 | 270 | 6 | 32 | 6 | 30 | ___ | ___ |
| 11 | 85 | 21 | 167 | 9 | 42 | 3 | 14 | ___ | ___ |
| 7 | 58 | 9 | 54 | 7 | 25 | 4 | 15 | ___ | ___ |
| 4 | 14 | 9 | 64 | 7 | 28 | 6 | 23 | ___ | ___ |
| 6 | 56 | 31 | 194 | 5 | 25 | 3 | 19 | ___ | ___ |
| 5 | 30 | 30 | 260 | 2 | 7 | 2 | 6 | ___ | ___ |
| 9 | 52 | 23 | 197 | 10 | 33 | 6 | 26 | ___ | ___ |
| 6 | 38 | 28 | 304 | 12 | 62 | 10 | 54 | ___ | ___ |
| 5 | 49 | 24 | 156 | 6 | 28 | 7 | 37 | ___ | ___ |
| 4 | 25 | 15 | 110 | 14 | 50 | 11 | 45 | ___ | ___ |

| Total Patients | Total Days | ALOS | Total ALOS |
|---|---|---|---|
| Med _____ | Med _____ | Med _____ | _____ |
| Surg _____ | Surg _____ | Surg _____ | |
| OB _____ | OB _____ | OB _____ | |
| NB _____ | NB _____ | NB _____ | |

**G. Compute the LOS based on the following information:**

| Month | Discharges | Days | ALOS |
|---|---|---|---|
| January | 142 | 794 | _____ |
| February | 137 | 872 | _____ |
| March | 155 | 832 | _____ |
| April | 162 | 955 | _____ |
| May | 154 | 787 | _____ |
| June | 148 | 585 | _____ |
| July | 159 | 667 | _____ |
| August | 164 | 702 | _____ |
| September | 155 | 699 | _____ |
| October | 165 | 790 | _____ |
| November | 150 | 682 | _____ |
| December | 122 | 502 | _____ |
| **Totals** | _____ | _____ | _____ |

## H. Monthly statistics:

**2000 Annual Statistics**

| | |
|---|---|
| Inpatient discharges | (Total) |
|     Adults and Children | 10810 |
|     Newborn | 1601 |
| Inpatient discharges by Clinical Service | |
|     Medicine | 6050 |
|     Surgical | 2828 |
|     Obstetric | 1932 |
| Service Days | |
|     Adults and Children | 60420 |
|     Newborn | 4623 |
| Discharge Days (Total) | |
|     Adults and Children | 73104 |
|     Newborn | 4808 |
| Discharge Days (Service) | |
|     Medicine | 36500 |
|     Surgical | 31708 |
|     Obstetrics | 4896 |
| Births | 1615 |
| Deliveries | 1640 |
| Operations | 1005 |

1. What is the ALOS for Adults and Children? _____
2. What is the ALOS for Newborns? _____
3. What is the ALOS for each clinical service?
   Medicine _____
   Surgical _____
   Obstetrics _____

## 8-4: THOUGHT QUESTIONS

1. What is the function of a hypothesis? Explain the difference between a null hypothesis and an alternative hypothesis.
2. Explain the meaning of a p-value. Why does the p-value have to be small in order for the null hypothesis to be rejected?
3. A researcher carried out a significance test and found that the p-value associated with the computed test statistic was .032. If the researcher had chosen a .01 significance level, would the null hypothesis be rejected? What if the researcher had chosen a .05 significance level?
4. How is sample size related to the probability of Type II error?
5. What is the purpose of interval estimation?
6. Pairs of variables are given below. Indicate whether you would expect the relationship between the variables in each pair to be positive or negative and support your answer.
   A. the number of beds in a hospital and the number of employees in a hospital
   B. the age of a car and its resale value
   C. students' high school QPAs and their college QPAs
   D. the amount of computer experience students have had and their degree of confidence in using computers
   E. the number of prescription medications taken by adults and their self-rating of their health on a scale of 1 to 10, with 1 meaning extremely poor health and 10 meaning excellent health
7. A HIM professional reads the following statement in a journal article: "In a sample of 823 clerical workers a significant relationship was found between their scores on the XYZ Clerical Aptitude Test and their job performance ratings by their supervisors (Pearson correlation coefficient = .15, p = .009)." The HIM professional concludes that there must be a very strong relationship between the aptitude test and job performance. Do you agree with this conclusion? Why or why not?
8. The office manager at a medical practice reviews a random sample of insurance forms prepared over the past year and finds that 8% of the forms contain errors. She constructs a 95% confidence interval for the population proportion. The lower and upper limits of the confidence interval are 3% and 13% respectively. If all the insurance forms were reviewed rather than only a sample, is it possible that more than 13% would contain errors? Explain your answer.

Copyright © 2001 by W.B. Saunders Company. All rights reserved.

## 8-5: TYPE I OR TYPE II ERROR

### Assignment:

*A researcher is interested in comparing two local hospitals. He studies a random sample of the records of patients admitted to each hospital under a particular DRG within a designated time period. Four hypothetical scenarios are given below. The following information is provided for each scenario: the null hypothesis being tested, the decision reached by the researcher on the basis of a test of significance, and the true status of the population. For each scenario determine whether the researcher has made a correct decision, a Type I error, or a Type II error. Support your answer.*

A. **Scenario 1**

   Null hypothesis: There is no difference in the average length of stay in Hospital A and Hospital B.

   Decision: Fail to reject the null hypothesis

   Status of population: The average length of stay is longer in Hospital B than in Hospital A.

B. **Scenario 2**

   Null hypothesis: There is no difference in the average charges in Hospital A and Hospital B.

   Decision: Reject the null hypothesis.

   Status of population: The average charges are higher in Hospital B than in Hospital A.

C. **Scenario 3**

   Null hypothesis: There is no difference in the average ages of patients treated at Hospital A and Hospital B.

   Decision: Reject the null hypothesis.

   Status in population: The average ages of patients treated at Hospital A and Hospital B are the same.

D. **Scenario 4**

   Null hypothesis: There is no difference in the average number of patients treated at Hospital A and Hospital B.

   Decision: Fail to reject the null hypothesis.

   Status of population: On the average an equal number of patients are treated at Hospital A and Hospital B.

## 8-6: RESEARCH ARTICLE

### Assignment:

*Find an article in an HIM journal that reports the results of one of the tests of significance discussed in this chapter. Answer the following questions regarding the test of significance.*

    A.  Which significance test was used?
    B.  State the hypothesis that was tested.
    C.  State the level of significance that was used.
    D.  Was the null hypothesis rejected?
    E.  What conclusions were made by the author(s) on the basis of the significance test? Do these conclusions seem consistent with the results of the test?

# Review Answers

## PRETEST REVIEW ANSWER KEY

### Directions:

1. Correct your Pretest answers with the answers below by placing a slash through the incorrect question number (Example: 8) with a pen or pencil of a contrasting color.
2. Record the correct answer by placing a square around the letter of the correct answer.
3. Record the total correct on the Initial Performance Grid in Section 4 of this review manual.
4. Calculate your performance rate and also record on the grid.
5. Promptly locate the correct answer for each question missed in the chapter of the textbook.
6. Proceed to the chapter review if your performance rate was 80% or higher; otherwise, return to the chapter for further study.

### Answers to Pretest Review:

| 1.  | a | 6.  | a |
| --- | --- | --- | --- |
| 2.  | b | 7.  | b |
| 3.  | a | 8.  | a |
| 4.  | b | 9.  | a |
| 5.  | a | 10. | a |

## CHAPTER REVIEW ANSWER KEY

### Directions:

1. Correct your answers with the answers below by placing a slash through the incorrect question number (Example: 8) with a pen or pencil of a contrasting color.
2. Record the correct answer by placing a square around the letter of the correct answer.
3. Record the total correct on the Initial Performance Grid in Section 4 of this review manual.
4. Calculate your performance rate and also record on the grid.
5. Promptly locate the correct answer for each question missed in the chapter of the textbook.
6. Proceed to the next chapter assigned in your study.

### Answers to Chapter Review:

| 1. | a | 6.  | a |
| --- | --- | --- | --- |
| 2. | b | 7.  | d |
| 3. | c (10 x 100) / (51 - 2) | 8.  | b (1, 2, 4, 7, 8, 11, 22) |
| 4. | a | 9.  | c (22 - 1) = 21 |
| 5. | b | 10. | 11.8 days (20 + 10 + 7 + 14 + 8) / 5 |

Copyright © 2001 by W.B. Saunders Company. All rights reserved.

# CHAPTER 9

# RESEARCH AND EPIDEMIOLOGY

## Review

### PRETEST REVIEW

**Directions:**

1. Read each question carefully before selecting an answer.
2. Circle the letter of the correct answer.
3. Answer all the questions since there is no penalty for this pretest review.
4. Check your answers with the answer key located at the end of this chapter.

1. The ability of a test instrument to measure what it is supposed to measure is called:
   a. validity
   b. reliability
   c. agreement
   d. kappa statistic

2. The study of disease and determinants of disease in populations is called:
   a. clinical trial
   b. outcomes study
   c. epidemiology
   d. clinical medicine

3. Once the hypothesis is established, the second step of a good research study is to conduct a:
   a. preliminary study
   b. selection of subjects
   c. review of IRB rules
   d. literature review

4. The specific aims should include the project's _____ and should be both _____ and _____.
   a. goals or objectives; short and long term
   b. end results or conclusions; succinct and clear
   c. hypothesis; explicit and concise
   d. budget; salaries and equipment

5. Which section of the research proposal should include the importance of the research project supported by a review of past research studies (literature review) and preliminary research performed by the author?
   a. methodology
   b. significance
   c. specific aims
   d. hypothesis

6. Which section of the research proposal includes such things as: data collection process, IRB application, statisical analysis of the data, time frame, sample size, place of study?
   a. procedures
   b. process
   c. significance
   d. methodology

7. Informed consent, confidentiality, risks and benefits of people enrolled in the study, and the demographic description of the subjects are all included in which section of the research proposal?
   a. human subjects
   b. appendix
   c. literature cited
   d. specific aims

8. Which type of study design modifies the health characteristics that are found to cause the disease by using health care interventions that control the disease from progressing or prevent the disease from occurring?
   a. analytic study
   b. descriptive study
   c. outcomes study
   d. experimental study

9. Which type of study design is normally used to generate hypotheses?
   a. analytic study
   b. experimental study
   c. descriptive study
   d. none of the above

10. Which statistic is an estimate of the relative risk—is used in case-control studies, when the disease under study is rare, and when cases are true representatives of all cases and controls?
    a. odds ratio
    b. life analysis
    c. correlation
    d. regression

# CHAPTER REVIEW

## Directions:

1. *Read each question carefully before selecting an answer.*
2. *Circle the letter of the correct answer.*
3. *Answer all the questions since there is no penalty for this pretest review.*
4. *Check your answers with the answer key located at the end of this chapter.*

1. One disadvantage of this type of epidemiological study design is that it only examines survivors and those living as cases. It is called a:
   a. clinical trial
   b. community trial
   c. prospective study
   d. cross-sectional prevalence study

2. Which study design is well suited for rare diseases or those diseases with a long latency period such as cancer and heart disease?
   a. prospective study
   b. clinical trial
   c. descriptive study
   d. case-control study

3. Which type of life analysis is appropriate for both large and small sample sizes and provides a survival curve as a method to examine survival among two different groups?
   a. Rank and Survival Method
   b. Kaplan-Meier Product Limit Method
   c. Standardized Mortality Method
   d. Censorship and Survival Method

4. What is the reproducibility (or reliability) between more than one research assistant or observer called?
   a. intraobserver reliability
   b. interobserver reliability
   c. bias
   d. consistency

5. When selecting subjects for a research study, researchers are more likely to choose people who are frequently under medical care. What type of bias is this called?
   a. survival bias
   b. diagnosis bias
   c. selection bias
   d. recall bias

6. Subjects with faulty memory, or who tend to remember certain types of information because of their exposure or the disease under study, leads to what type of bias?
   a. nonresponse bias
   b. recall bias
   c. prevarication bias
   d. sampling variability

7. Which method reduces interviewer bias?
   a. provide intensive training for the interviewers
   b. standardize the interview form
   c. a & b
   d. a only

8. In a case-control study, why are the cases and controls often matched on variables such as age and sex?
   a. so that cases and controls are similar except for the disease and health characteristic under study
   b. so that cases and controls are similar for all aspects of the study
   c. so that cases and controls are similar except for the disease under study only
   d. so that cases and controls are similar except for the health characteristic only

9. What is a tentative assertion called that is assumed by the researcher but not positively known until it is tested?
   a. significance
   b. hypothesis
   c. methodology
   d. specific aims

10. The incidence rate of the exposed group divided by the incidence rate of the unexposed group is the formula used to determine:
    a. relative risk
    b. odds ratio
    c. incidence
    d. prevalence

*Additional review questions can be found on the CD-ROM.*

# Assignments

## 9-1: THOUGHT QUESTIONS

1. The research plan is a very important part of the entire research proposal development. List the components of the research proposal that make up the research plan.
2. A researcher would like to determine the effectiveness of a new radiology test in detecting multi-infarct dementia. The specificity rate was found to be 88% and the sensitivity rate was 94%. Do you believe this new radiology test is valid? Why or why not?
3. Describe the Kappa statistic.
    A. What is a Kappa statistic and when should it be used?
    B. What is a good standard value for this statistic?
    C. If your Kappa statistic was 0.40, what would you conclude?
4. Describe the prospective study design.
    A. Why is the prospective study design the best analytical design to use?
    B. What steps are included in a typical prospective study?
5. Compare the prospective study design to the historical-prospective study design.
    A. What is the major difference between the prospective study design and the historical-prospective study design?
    B. What is the major advantage of the historical-prospective study design when compared with the prospective study design?
6. Describe Life-Table Analysis.
    A. What is a person-time denominator and when is it used?
    B. What are the assumptions that must be met before using life table analysis?
    C. For which study designs are life table analysis most appropriate?

## 9-2: THE SIGNIFICANCE OF LITERATURE IN RESEARCH STUDIES

### Assignment:

*Conduct a literature search and compose the literature review and significance sections of the research study.*

1. Choose an HIM related topic.
2. Conduct a literature search on the topic chosen using the databases available in the library such as Medline, etc. The reference librarian is an excellent resource to provide instruction in using these databases.
3. Collect and review articles.
4. Write the literature review and significance sections showing the need and importance of doing research in this area.

## 9-3: THE INSTITUTIONAL REVIEW BOARD

### Scenario:

A researcher has requested to study the cause of atrial fibrillation using patient medical records. The proposal states that the collection of patient identifying information such as patient name, address, etc. is not needed.

  A. Is it necessary to submit this research proposal to the Institutional Review Board of the hospital where the data will be collected? Explain your answer.
  B. What is an IRB and what is its primary purpose?
  C. Why is the IRB so important in the review of proposed research studies?

## 9-4: RESEARCH BUDGET

### Assignment:

*For a research proposal to study the prevalence of electronic health records (EHR) systems in health care facilities across the country, what items would be included in the budget? Provide an approximate cost for each item.*

## 9-5: HIM USE OF DESCRIPTIVE RESEARCH

*The Director of Health Information Services and Systems at Anywhere Health Care is responsible for determining whether a state-of-the-art patient encounter system is appropriate for the facility. Using a descriptive study, the Director would first like to determine how many facilities in the country actually use an on-line patient encounter system.*

  A. Would this study also be considered a prevalence study? Why or why not?
  B. Describe a prevalence study.
  C. What is the difference between point prevalence and period prevalence?
  D. Describe the method used to collect data for this type of study. Justify your selection of this method of data collection.

## 9-6: CASE CONTROL STUDY

### Assignment:

*Using a case-control study design, test the following hypothesis:*

Hypothesis: No physical activity (walking, jogging, light aerobics, etc.) during pregnancy can lead to delivery by C-section.

Specify the following for the study:

1. Cases and controls: description of population to be included in each
2. Method for obtaining cases and controls
3. Data collection methodology
4. Data to be collected
5. Sample Size
6. Confounding variables
7. Statistical tests to be used

## 9-7: RESEARCH STUDY DESIGNS

### Assignment:

*For each of the following scenarios, determine the type of research study design to be used.*

1. Using patient records of women who were diagnosed with COPD in 1960, determine whether they were exposed to smoking (personal or passive). Follow them forward and determine their incidence of lung cancer and their survival status.
2. Identify a group of children with leukemia that is currently in remission and follow them forward for 20 years to determine their risk of other cancers and their survival status.
3. Identify individuals with rheumatoid arthritis (cases) and individuals without rheumatoid arthritis (controls). Interview both cases and controls to determine their past and present diets and specific foods most frequently eaten, such as milk, fruit, etc.
4. Identify all cases of HIV infection within a specific community.
5. Select a group of individuals with Alzheimer's disease. Randomize into three groups—one group will be treated with drug A, one group will be treated with drug B, and the third group will be treated with a placebo. Follow all groups forward for the next 5 years to determine improvement/decline in the disease.

## 9-8: ANALYSIS OF RESEARCH METHODOLOGIES

1. Using a current article on HIM research, determine the study hypothesis, methodology, and statistical analysis. Identify the following in the article:
   A. study hypothesis
   B. study design
   C. study methodology
   D. statistical tests utilized
   E. conclusions
   F. types of bias in the study

2. Explain how the study could be performed differently or more appropriately in order to test a similar hypothesis. Include in the explanation:
   A. New study hypothesis (if it is different from the original study)
   B. New study design
   C. New study methodology regarding what would change: sample size, data collection methods, data sources, etc.
   D. Different statistical tests—specify why they were chosen and how they may be more appropriate in order to test the hypothesis
   E. Study limitations

## 9-9: EPIDEMIOLOGY AND HIM

### Assignment:

*Using epidemiological study design and the following sample, develop a research study hypotheses related to one of the following health information management functions that includes the same components as the sample.*

1. Release of information/correspondence
2. Transcription
3. Utilization review/management
4. Quality assessment and improvement
5. Record analysis/quantitative analysis
6. Record retention
7. Record retrieval
8. Coding

#### Sample Epidemiology Design for HIM

**Purpose:** Determine if there was a relationship between years as a transcriptionist and the development of Carpal Tunnel Syndrome (CTS).

**Hypothesis:** Transcriptionists working more than 5 years will have an increased incidence of CTS.

**Study Design:** Prospective/Cohort/Incidence Study

**Methodology:** Study group (transcribing for > 5 years) and comparison group (not transcriptionists) and follow them forward in time to determine the incidence of CTS.

**Statistical analysis:** Incidence rates, relative risk, and survival analysis or survival curves. Medical exams will be performed on both groups at the beginning of the study and yearly thereafter to test for development of CTS.

## 9-10: DATA COLLECTION

*Data has been collected on the completeness of the surgical informed consent. Over 200 records have been reviewed for the presence of the following data items on the consent form:*

- Date and time the consent was completed and explained to the patient;
- Type of surgery performed;
- Risks and/or possible complications of surgery;
- Patient's signature, date, time of signing
- Physician/surgeon's signature, date, time of signing
- Witness/nurse's signature, date, time of signing

Explain the following:
  A. Set up a database or spreadsheet to show how data will be collected: show column heads and the methods for recording presence or absence of data item on the consent form.
  B. What software would you use to organize the data? Why would this be the best software for this project?
  C. How would you tabulate your findings? List the descriptive statistics that would be used.
  D. Would you use any additional software to further analyze the data?

## 9-11: DATA ANALYSIS

*On the CD is an Access database entitled "Defense" that includes financial and clinical data on 165 patients. The data includes the following items:*

1. Date of admission
2. DRG and weight of the DRG
3. Length of stay
4. Cost of the stay
5. DRG payment or reimbursement amount
6. Total payment (which includes more than the DRG payment because it may include additional amounts for the hospital since it is a teaching hospital, etc.)
7. + OR – (total payment—cost of the stay)
8. Infect (total infections)
9. Nosocomial infections (those infections acquired 72 hours after admission)
10. Community-acquired infections (those infections acquired less than 72 hours after admission)

Answer the following questions using queries to the Defense database.

A. Number of infections and cost of care
B. Number of infections and DRG reimbursement
C. Number of infections and total payment or reimbursement
D. Type of infection and cost of care
E. Type of DRG, number of infections, and cost of care
F. Type of DRG, type of infection, and profit or loss for the hospital
G. At least two additional queries of your own

## 9-12: PROSPECTIVE STUDY ON DATA TRENDS

*Design a prospective study that would further analyze a trend or pattern from the Defense database. Complete the following steps to complete this assignment.*

1. Choose a trend from the defense database
2. Formulate a hypothesis
3. State your specific aims
4. Establish the research methodology
5. Discuss what statistical tests should be done to test your hypothesis

# Review Answers

## PRETEST REVIEW ANSWER KEY

### Directions:

1. Correct your Pretest answers with the answers below by placing a slash through the incorrect question number (Example: 8) with a pen or pencil of a contrasting color.
2. Record the correct answer by placing a square around the letter of the correct answer.
3. Record the total correct on the Initial Performance Grid in Section 4 of this review manual.
4. Calculate your performance rate and also record on the grid.
5. Promptly locate the correct answer for each question missed in the chapter of the textbook.
6. Proceed to the chapter review if your performance rate was 80% or higher; otherwise, return to the chapter for further study.

### Answers to Pretest Review:

| | | | |
|---|---|---|---|
| 1. | a | 6. | d |
| 2. | c | 7. | a |
| 3. | d | 8. | d |
| 4. | a | 9. | c |
| 5. | b | 10. | a |

## CHAPTER REVIEW ANSWER KEY

### Directions:

1. Correct your answers with the answers below by placing a slash through the incorrect question number (Example: 8) with a pen or pencil of a contrasting color.
2. Record the correct answer by placing a square around the letter of the correct answer.
3. Record the total correct on the Initial Performance Grid in Section 4 of this review manual.
4. Calculate your performance rate and also record on the grid.
5. Promptly locate the correct answer for each question missed in the chapter of the textbook.
6. Proceed to the next chapter assigned in your study.

### Answers to Chapter Review:

| | | | |
|---|---|---|---|
| 1. | d | 6. | b |
| 2. | d | 7. | c |
| 3. | b | 8. | a |
| 4. | b | 9. | b |
| 5. | c | 10. | a |

# CHAPTER 10

# QUALITY MANAGEMENT AND CLINICAL OUTCOMES

## Review

### PRETEST REVIEW

### Directions:

1. Read each question carefully before selecting an answer.
2. Circle the letter of the correct answer.
3. Answer all the questions since there is no penalty for this pretest review.
4. Check your answers with the answer key located at the end of this chapter.

1. Five years is the contract period for each PRO Scope of Work.
   a. True
   b. False

2. The National Practitioner Data Bank maintains data on the actions of state licensing boards.
   a. True
   b. False

3. The Office of Fiscal and Budgetary Management has jurisdiction over peer review organizations.
   a. True
   b. False

4. Medical record review by the medical staff of the documentation practices of staff physicians is required by the JCAHO to be an ongoing process.
   a. True
   b. False

5. Processing reimbursement claims for inpatient services provided to Medicare beneficiaries is the function of the fiscal intermediary.
   a. True
   b. False

6. Report of a potentially compensable event is to risk management as a patient's discharge plan is to utilization management.
   a. True
   b. False

7. Medical staff credentialing is a general function of the medical records committee.
   a. True
   b. False

8. Outlier data points are associated with DRG reimbursement.
   a. True
   b. False

9. For hospitals, the *Conditions of Participation* detail regulations governing provider services to Medicare and Medicaid patients.
   a. True
   b. False

10. Every state, by law, protects information generated under peer review processes.
    a. True
    b. False

## CHAPTER REVIEW

### Directions:

1. Read each question carefully before selecting an answer.
2. Circle the letter of the correct answer.
3. Answer all the questions since there is no penalty for this pretest review.
4. Check your answers with the answer key located at the end of this chapter.

1. The Donabedian Model of Structure, Process and Outcome is conceptualized around three domains that include:
   a. amenities
   b. interpersonal
   c. technological
   d. both b and c

2. Which of the following performance evaluation measures examines interaction between patients and providers?
   a. outcome
   b. process
   c. structure
   d. none of the above

3. A quality indicator is an objective, quantifiable measurement that targets events, or patterns of events, suggestive of a problematic process or behavior.
   a. True
   b. False

4. A sentinel event is a frequently occurring undesirable outcome warranting further investigation.
   a. True
   b. False

5. When a criterion accurately measures the intended outcome of care and discriminates correctly between the presence and absence of the outcome, it is said to be:
   a. reliable
   b. valid
   c. both reliable and valid
   d. statistically significant

6. Renewing admissions, for example the principal diagnosis, is an evaluation function of the utilization review program.
   a. True
   b. False

7. Hospitals participating in the Medicare program would find directives regarding required quality assurance activities for Medicare published in all of the following except:
   a. Accreditation Manual for Hospitals
   b. Conditions of Participation
   c. Federal Register
   d. PRO Scope of Work

8. Targeted processes and outcomes mandated for quality review by the JCAHO include:
   a. high-risk processes
   b. high-volume processes
   c. problem-prone processes
   d. all of the above

9. The principal objective of a risk management program is the efficient management of claims against the health care facility.

   a. True
   b. False

10. The ultimate authority for making appointments and granting physician privileges is vested in the:

    a. credentialing committee
    b. executive committee
    c. governing body
    d. chief executive office

*Additional review questions can be found on the CD-ROM.*

# Assignments

## 10-1: INTERNET SCAVENGER HUNT

### Directions:

*Utilizing the Internet, answer the following questions on a separate piece of paper.*

*In your answers, specify the website name (URL and site name) where you found the answer. If desirable print the page with the answer. Your answer must be in your own words; reference to the printed page or copying the answer from the web will receive no credit. The terms in bold refer to the website where information is available.*

1. **Quality Management Professionals**

   A. Describe the mechanism **AHIMA** uses to serve HIM professionals who work in Quality Management (hint: specialty groups). What is the purpose of this group? What are the membership requirements?

   B. What is the certification for individuals who are experienced in quality assessment and improvement available from the **National Association for Healthcare Quality**? Name the credential and list the requirements needed to sit for the examination.

2. **Outcome Measures**

   A. Explain the purpose of the **Joint Commission's** ORYX initiative. What benefits are gained by integrating performance measures into the accreditation process? How does ORYX affect a Health Care Organization's (HCO) accreditation status? Explain the concepts and purposes of a performance measurement system and core measures. List a specific example of each.

   B. Describe and explain the purpose of HEDIS that is collected as part of **National Committee on Quality Assurance (NCQA)** accreditation. Give a specific example of a measure that is collected as part of HEDIS. What data items would provide evidence of this measure?

3. **Information Available to the Consumer**

   A. Identify the information available from the **Joint Commission** about a named accredited health care organization/facility. Do you feel this information is helpful to the consumer? Why or why not?

   B. Access an Accreditation Summary report from the **NCQA** for a managed health care plan that you are familiar with. For example: Exclusive HealthCare, Inc. is Mutual of Omaha's HMO; HMO Nebraska is Blue Cross of Nebraska's HMO. List the company name and its current accreditation status. What are areas of concern, e.g., a low score or less than full compliance?

Copyright © 2001 by W.B. Saunders Company. All rights reserved.

4. **Resources for Developing Quality Improvement Studies**

   A. Select a Clinical Practice Guideline developed by the **Agency for Healthcare Quality and Research.** List the topic. Identify and print a portion of the Guidelines that could be used to develop a quality improvement study. For this portion, identify the group of professionals who would use that study e.g., orthopedic physicians, physical therapists, and the group of patients by diagnosis, procedure, or other characteristic to be studied.

   B. Identify a disease or medical procedure. Search the web to identify sources of information for the consumer who has the disease, the health care professional who works with patients who have the disease, and information to use in a quality improvement study.

## 10-2: PEER REVIEW ORGANIZATION INFORMATION ON THE WEB

1. Find the website address (URL) for your state's peer review organization (PRO).
2. Perform research at the website and gather information about the following:
   A. Purpose of the organization
   B. Services provided by the organization, with special emphasis on the following:
      1. Quality improvement projects
      2. Utilization review
      3. Credentials verification
      4. Educational workshops for HIM professionals
      5. Professional services offered to health care facilities
      6. Publications
      7. Other contracts/special projects the PRO is engaged in
3. Prepare a written report based on the research done at the PRO website. The report should detail the purpose of the PRO and describe how the PRO contributes to a hospital's Quality Management Program.
4. Construct a table using word processing or spreadsheet software that displays the services provided by the PRO, a brief explanation of the service, and the type of health care professional who performs the service (i.e., physician, HIM professional, nurse, etc). Attach the table to the written report.

## 10-3: DATA COLLECTION ON PATIENT FALLS

### Directions:

1. Conduct a literature search to identify journal articles about patient falls in health care organizations. The search should focus on causes of falls (both clinical and environmental), staff and institutional responses to falls, suggestions for preventing falls, risk assessment techniques, environmental factors contributing to falls.
2. Prepare an annotated bibliography of relevant articles.
3. Design a data collection form based on information derived from the literature.
4. Using the form from number 3, abstract data from patient records.
5. Prepare a summary report of data analysis, including recommendations.

## 10-4: PROBLEM IDENTIFICATION USING PARETO ANALYSIS

*A local health information management (HIM) department has collected the following data on unfiled loose documents.*

### Directions:

1. Compute the percentages for the reasons not filed.
2. On either graph paper or using computer software, construct a Pareto diagram, stratified by reason not filed.

| Terminal Digit Section | Number Sampled | Documents Not Filed | Patient Number Missing | Wrong Patient Number | Record Not in Shelves | Wrong Patient Name | Other |
|---|---|---|---|---|---|---|---|
| 04 | 18 | 6 | 1 | 1 | 4 | 0 | 0 |
| 13 | 21 | 11 | 0 | 4 | 6 | 0 | 1 |
| 17 | 19 | 8 | 1 | 5 | 2 | 0 | 0 |
| 21 | 33 | 16 | 1 | 5 | 7 | 1 | 2 |
| 22 | 50 | 14 | 2 | 1 | 8 | 1 | 2 |
| 30 | 31 | 9 | 2 | 2 | 4 | 1 | 0 |
| 43 | 31 | 21 | 3 | 3 | 9 | 3 | 3 |
| 50 | 36 | 12 | 6 | 1 | 2 | 0 | 3 |
| 70 | 43 | 15 | 6 | 0 | 7 | 0 | 2 |
| 76 | 17 | 5 | 0 | 4 | 1 | 0 | 0 |
| 81 | 30 | 15 | 1 | 3 | 9 | 2 | 0 |
| 82 | 9 | 0 | 0 | 0 | 0 | 0 | 0 |
| 96 | 53 | 15 | 6 | 2 | 5 | 1 | 1 |
| 98 | 14 | 9 | 3 | 1 | 4 | 0 | 1 |
| 99 | 57 | 28 | 5 | 6 | 13 | 3 | 1 |
| Totals | 462 | 184 | 37 | 38 | 81 | 12 | 16 |
| Percentage of total errors | | | | | | | |

## 10-5: QUALITY MONITORING IN HIM

*A hospital has established the quality indicators listed below for the correspondence section. Data for the most recent review are provided.*

### Review of the Correspondence Section

| Indicator | Number of Requests Reviewed | Number of Errors | Error Rate |
|---|---|---|---|
| Nonrequested documents copied | 78 | 4 | |
| Requested documents not copied | 78 | 6 | |
| Poor quality of copies (i.e., smudged, off-sheet) | 78 | 23 | |
| Nonvalid authorization honored | 78 | 0 | |
| Poor quality of reassembly | 78 | 18 | |
| Turn-around > 3 working days | 78 | 3 | |
| Page count missing | 78 | 12 | |
| Incorrect billing | 78 | 8 | |
| Total | | 74 | |

### Directions:

1. Calculate the error rate for each indicator and a gross error rate. (Round to two decimal places.)
2. On graph paper or using computer software, construct a Pareto chart showing the indicators most often failed.
3. Brainstorm at least 10 possible reasons for the errors, remembering the philosophy "blame the process not the people."
4. Construct a fishbone diagram using the ideas from number 3 to display the possible causes.
5. In a narrative, discuss the findings from these diagrams and rates. What do these rates suggest? Are there any management implications? What recommendations would you make to the supervisor of the correspondence section?

## 10-6: USING RUN CHARTS TO TACKLE THE RECORD DELINQUENCY PROBLEM

### Scenario:

A corporate HIM director, for a major health care system, is preparing for a meeting with her four HIM supervisors. Each supervisor has delegated managerial responsibility for the HIM services in an acute care facility that is a part of the health care system. One important topic on the meeting agenda is the annual review of medical record delinquency rates for each facility. Two of the four facilities continue to struggle with rates that exceed JCAHO's allowable rate. The corporate director wants to distribute a graph that can be utilized for both comparison and benchmarking purposes.

### Directions:

1. Using spreadsheet software and the information presented in the tables below, calculate a monthly medical record delinquency rate for each of the four facilities. In addition, calculate the yearly average delinquency rate for each site. Construct a run chart that displays this information in pictorial form. The run chart should have a legend that accurately identifies each facility.
2. Assume the role of one of the HIM supervisors. Brainstorm methods for decreasing the delinquency rates in the facilities that are not in compliance with JCAHO standards for medical records completion. Submit a list of suggestions that would help to improve medical record delinquency rates.

| Month | Average Monthly Discharges | | | |
|---|---|---|---|---|
| | Hospital A | Hospital B | Hospital C | Hospital D |
| January | 1289 | 803 | 980 | 630 |
| February | 1178 | 784 | 965 | 610 |
| March | 1089 | 798 | 1023 | 598 |
| April | 1110 | 692 | 923 | 539 |
| May | 1256 | 730 | 1114 | 605 |
| June | 987 | 710 | 1002 | 628 |
| July | 1032 | 690 | 945 | 560 |
| August | 921 | 640 | 969 | 520 |
| September | 1125 | 720 | 1164 | 578 |
| October | 1343 | 754 | 1049 | 649 |
| November | 1378 | 780 | 1156 | 673 |
| December | 1253 | 775 | 1041 | 621 |

| Month | Number of Delinquent Medical Records | | | |
|---|---|---|---|---|
| | Hospital A | Hospital B | Hospital C | Hospital D |
| January | 734 | 303 | 367 | 429 |
| February | 685 | 276 | 379 | 459 |
| March | 621 | 245 | 391 | 427 |
| April | 687 | 202 | 303 | 402 |
| May | 743 | 240 | 387 | 469 |
| June | 785 | 189 | 413 | 473 |
| July | 679 | 169 | 393 | 410 |
| August | 623 | 174 | 381 | 398 |
| September | 713 | 190 | 402 | 419 |
| October | 825 | 204 | 382 | 438 |
| November | 745 | 213 | 374 | 441 |
| December | 798 | 198 | 389 | 414 |

## 10-7: GROUP PROJECT: SYSTEM EFFECTS

*This assignment demonstrates the system effects on process and illustrates system constraints that cause bottlenecks and impede productivity.*

### Players:

Chief Operations Officer (productivity driver/timekeeper)
Chief Information Officer (motivator)
Discharge Planner (die roller - controls input)
Clerk—logs discharge records into locator system
Clerk—assembles records in correct filing order
Clerk—analyzes records for completeness
Clerk—codes diagnoses on records

### Materials needed:

Stopwatch or timer
Die
Small containers for each clerk (salad bowls will work)
Paper clips, coins, or buttons to simulate records (50–75)

### Directions:

Workers are given "job descriptions" and instructed that the production process is sequential. The COO sets a productivity goal, the number of "records" to be processed in three minutes, and begins the time count. The discharge planner rolls the die and begins system input; each roll of the die determines the number of "records" which move to the next step of the process. The COO continually pressures the workers to meet their goal, to work faster, and reports time left at intervals. The CIO encourages and praises the efforts of the workers to process "records."

### Discussion Questions:

The group will address the following issues:

1. How does CIO's encouragement and praise affect productivity?
2. How does the pressure from the COO affect productivity?
3. What key factors do affect productivity?
4. What should be done before the process is automated/computerized?
5. Who knows the most about improving the process?

## 10-8: GROUP PROJECT: THE "SIX LESSON" INSPECTION DEMONSTRATION

*As adapted by Dr. Joseph G. Van Matre, University of Alabama at Birmingham.*

### Directions:

1. Count the number of "e's" in the following paragraph.
2. Collect the number of "e's" reported by each member of the group. Plot the data to show variation.
3. Ask for a recount. Offer extra points on the final grade if the count is "correct."
4. Have each member report the number counted and plot again.
5. Ask group members for suggestions to decrease the variability in count.
6. Have each student report the number counted and plot again.
7. Discuss lessons learned.

### Inspection Demonstration Document

"Business and other human endeavors are also systems. They, too, are bound by invisible fabrics of interrelated actions, which often take years to fully play out their effects on each other. Since we are part of that lacework ourselves, it's doubly hard to see the whole pattern of change. Instead, we tend to focus on snapshots of isolated parts of the system, and wonder why our deepest problems never seem to get solved. System thinking is a conceptual framework, a body of knowledge and tools that has been developed over the past fifty years, to make the full patterns clearer, and to help us see how to change them effectively."

Peter Senge, *The Fifth Discipline*

## 10-9: STAKEHOLDER ANALYSIS AND MAPPING

Stakeholder analysis is a technique for identifying individuals, groups, and organizations with a stake in the decisions and actions of an organization. As some stakeholders are customers, the stakeholder map tool also may be useful in assessing customer relations.

Internal stakeholders are individuals or groups who operate almost entirely inside the organization (or inside the department), such as managers, professionals, and staff.

External stakeholders are individuals, groups, or companies outside the organization (or outside the department) who have an interest in the department. External stakeholders may provide inputs to the department, thus a symbiotic relationship, such as information system vendors, or the Human Resources Department. Stakeholders also may be competitors or others with a special [individual] interest in the department's services, such as vendors that outsource HIM services, physicians' office personnel, or the medical/clinical staff.

The HIM Department should determine its "key" stakeholders, those who have the greatest stake in the department operations (cooperative or threatening), and use appropriate techniques for managing relationships with those stakeholders. Blair and Fottler (1990) describe a simple technique to identify strategies for managing stakeholders. Create a 2 x 2 matrix with threat potential (high & low) on one axis, and cooperation potential (high & low) on the other. Rate the stakeholder's potential for threat and for cooperation as either high or low. Generic strategies are identified for each of the four categories of stakeholders shown in the matrix. See the following examples of the matrix and generic strategies.

### Directions:

1. Brainstorm a list of stakeholders or customers for the HIM department.
2. Classify each stakeholder into one of the four categories and discuss appropriate management tactics.
3. Create a stakeholder map for the HIM department.

### Generic Stakeholder Management Strategies

*Potential for Threat*

|  | High | Low |
|---|---|---|
| **High** (Potential for Cooperation) | Mixed-blessing stakeholder | Supportive stakeholder |
| **Low** | Nonsupportive stakeholder | Marginal stakeholder |

**Generic Strategies:**

- Mixed-blessing stakeholders can become supportive or nonsupportive based on issue. Manage by collaboration tactics.
- Supportive stakeholders are the ideal. Manage by involving them in your projects.
- Nonsupportive stakeholders can make life difficult. Manage by defending against them.
- Marginal stakeholders are likely to matter only on specific issues. Manage by monitoring their interest in projects.

*Source: Adapted from Blair, J.D., & Fottler, M.D. (1990). Challenges in Health Care Management. San Francisco: Jossey-Bass.*

## 10-10: QUALITY IMPROVEMENT TOOLS

Developed by Michael Wiggins for use in the HIM Program at the University of Alabama at Birmingham. Used with permission.

### Directions:

*Read each scenario and determine the appropriate QI tool to analyze the data.*

### Scenario 1:

The Health Care Organization uses a contract agent for after-hours x-ray services. The film images are made at an off-site clinic. The ordering physician reads the image for immediate treatment needs, and forwards the film and preliminary report to the on-site radiologist. The radiologist looks for discrepancies and omitted findings, and sends a final report back to the ordering physician. The final report should be received within 72 hours. The data on this process are: 1) the number of after-hours procedures per month; 2) the number of final reports received within 72 hours per month; 3) the average turn-around time per month.

### Questions:

1. Which tool would best illustrate if a trend exists in the timing of receiving reports?
2. Develop a "dummy" of the above tool labeling each part.

### Scenario 2:

A new team has been created. Several different departments are represented, and team members don't know each other. Each department has a different perspective on the process to be studied.

### Question:

What tool will help everyone "get on the same page" and understand the process as it currently operates?

### Scenario 3:

The administrative manager of the perinatal intensive care unit (PICU) feels that the case managers are incorrect about the average length of stay (ALOS) in the PICU being 3.4 days. The manager is basing his "feelings" on his daily observations. The data from the past few months show that the case managers have calculated the ALOS correctly. The manager still thinks something is wrong, "feels" that the "typical" length of stay is shorter than 3.4 days, and suspects that the mean is not the appropriate measure to use. The manager has the length of stay data for every patient who has been discharged from the unit for the past year.

### Question:

What tool will better analyze the data to determine if the data set is skewed?

## Scenario 4:

The hospital finance officer reports that the health care organization is spending too much money replacing linens. No data are available about why linens are "lost." Gathering hard data on why linens are lost is impossible (if each piece of linen could be tracked, it wouldn't be lost).

## Question:

What tool will help you answer the question, "Why are we losing linens?"

## Scenario 5:

The hospital loses a lot of linen, but no one knows what type of linen (sheets, blankets, towels, etc.) is lost most frequently. As a starting point, data are collected on the amount of money spent replacing each type of linen.

## Question:

What tool will help focus on the most important issue?

## Scenario 6:

On the Diabetic Care Unit, monitoring of the patients' blood sugar levels help them to stay in control with proper diet, exercise, and medication. Blood sugar levels are collected on all patients on the Diabetic Care Unit four times each day.

## Question:

What tool will help to monitor the blood sugar levels for abnormal variations?

## Scenario 7:

The manager of a pediatric unit is concerned about the prescription orders for a particular medication. Generally, dosage orders for pediatric medications are based on the patient's weight.

## Question:

Which tool would help to see if there is or is not a correlation between patient weight and the prescribed dosage of this medication?

## 10-11: AVOIDING LIABILITY: PATIENT SAFETY

Developed by Patrice Spath for use in the HIM Program at the University of Alabama at Birmingham. Used with permission.

### Case Study: A Medication Error

A patient was admitted to the ICU for a cardiac-related problem. On admission to the unit, the doctor ordered "Inderal 20 mg orally q 6 hours. If patient cannot take PO medications, give 1mg Inderal IV q 6 hours." Later that day, the patient transferred to a step-down unit. As required by the hospital's policy, an ICU nurse rewrote the patient's orders prior to her transfer to the step-down unit. However, the initial order was miscopied as "Inderal 20 mg orally q 6 hours; if patient cannot take PO give Inderal IV."

Upon the patient's arrival in the step-down unit, the admitting nurse asked the unit clerk to call the pharmacy for additional ampules of intravenous Inderal because the unit did not have enough in floor stock to administer a 20 mg infusion. The unit clerk gave no information about the patient or the specific order to the pharmacist. The pharmacist questioned this request and found the following information about IV Inderal in the MICROMEDEX:

"The IV form of Inderal (propranolol) can be infused at a maximum rate of 2 to 3 mg per hour. In clinical practice, the amount of IV propranolol required to replace PO propranolol varies depending on individual pharmacokinetics and other clinical circumstances. An IV dose of 10% of the oral dose may be used temporarily to replace the oral dose in patients undergoing surgery."

Using the MICROMEDEX information as a guideline, the pharmacist talked with the patient's nurse and they agreed the patient should receive an infusion of 3 mg/hr. The pharmacy sent 30 1-mg propranolol ampules to the unit, and the nurse prepared an 18 mg (18 ampules) infusion to run in over 6 hours.

After receiving 24 mg of propranolol over approximately 8 hours, the patient's blood pressure dropped to 70/50 and she complained of dizziness. The infusion was stopped. The patient's physician was contacted. The patient was placed on a cardiac monitor and watched closely. Her symptoms eventually subsided. There were no apparent lasting effects of the medication error.

### Directions:

*Write a report that includes answers to the following questions:*

1. What departments should be represented on the root cause analysis team that investigates this patient incident?
2. What evidence should be presented to the root cause analysis team? Evidence includes written or verbal testimony, physical evidence, and documents. Be as specific as possible.
3. Based on your search of the literature and the recommendations from national and state organizations involved in reducing medication errors, what appear to be the root cause(s) of this event? Cite the references you used in selecting each root cause.
4. Based on your search of the literature and the recommendations from national and state organizations involved in reducing medication errors, what process changes need to occur at this hospital to prevent similar medication errors from occurring? Cite the references you used in selecting each of your process improvement recommendations.

Copyright © 2001 by W.B. Saunders Company. All rights reserved.

# Review Answers

## PRETEST REVIEW ANSWER KEY

### Directions:

1. Correct your Pretest answers with the answers below by placing a slash through the incorrect question number (Example: *8*) with a pen or pencil of a contrasting color.
2. Record the correct answer by placing a square around the letter of the correct answer.
3. Record the total correct on the Initial Performance Grid in Section 4 of this review manual.
4. Calculate your performance rate and also record on the grid.
5. Promptly locate the correct answer for each question missed in the chapter of the textbook.
6. Proceed to the chapter review if your performance rate was 80% or higher; otherwise, return to the chapter for further study.

### Answers to Pretest Review:

| | | | |
|---|---|---|---|
| 1. | b | 6. | a |
| 2. | a | 7. | b |
| 3. | b | 8. | a |
| 4. | b | 9. | a |
| 5. | a | 10. | a |

## CHAPTER REVIEW ANSWER KEY

### Directions:

1. Correct your answers with the answers below by placing a slash through the incorrect question number (Example: *8*) with a pen or pencil of a contrasting color.
2. Record the correct answer by placing a square around the letter of the correct answer.
3. Record the total correct on the Initial Performance Grid in Section 4 of this review manual.
4. Calculate your performance rate and also record on the grid.
5. Promptly locate the correct answer for each question missed in the chapter of the textbook.
6. Proceed to the next chapter assigned in your study.

### Answers to Chapter Review:

| | | | |
|---|---|---|---|
| 1. | d | 6. | a |
| 2. | b | 7. | a |
| 3. | a | 8. | d |
| 4. | b | 9. | b |
| 5. | b | 10. | c |

# CHAPTER 11

# HEALTH LAW CONCEPTS AND PRACTICES

## Review

### PRETEST REVIEW

### Directions:

1. *Read each question carefully before selecting an answer.*
2. *Circle the letter of the correct answer.*
3. *Answer all the questions since there is no penalty for this pretest review.*
4. *Check your answers with the answer key located at the end of this chapter.*

1. Medicare-certified alcohol and drug abuse facilities must comply with Regulations on Confidentiality of Alcohol and Drug Abuse Patient Records.

    a. True
    b. False

2. The right of privacy was granted by the U.S. Supreme Court in the Griswold v. Connecticut decision.

    a. True
    b. False

3. In a tort action, one party alleges that another party's wrongful conduct has caused him some harm.

    a. True
    b. False

4. In a contract action, one party alleges that an agreement existed between himself and another party, and that the other party has breached (broken) that agreement.

    a. True
    b. False

5. A claim against a health care facility for breach of confidentiality could be both a tort and a contract action.

    a. True
    b. False

6. The right of privacy is expressly guaranteed by the U.S. Constitution.

    a. True
    b. False

7. The plaintiff is the party who initiates a lawsuit.

    a. True
    b. False

8. The concept of respondeat superior refers to holding the employer, supervisor, or organization responsible for the actions or inactions of its employees or agents.

    a. True
    b. False

9. Defamation is an example of an intentional tort.

    a. True
    b. False

10. Injecting a patient with medicine against his wishes is an example of fraud.

    a. True
    b. False

## CHAPTER REVIEW

### Directions:

1. *Read each question carefully before selecting an answer.*
2. *Circle the letter of the correct answer.*
3. *Answer all the questions since there is no penalty for this pretest review.*
4. *Check your answers with the answer key located at the end of this chapter.*

1. The length of time health information must be maintained in some form is often dictated by record retention laws and regulations.
   a. True
   b. False

2. A health information professional can not be held liable for accidental destruction or loss of a patient's health information.
   a. True
   b. False

3. The U.S. Bill of Rights is a source of _____ law.

4. Rules and regulations of administrative agencies such as the DSHS are a source of law.
   a. True
   b. False

5. Invasion of privacy is a tort.
   a. True
   b. False

6. If the surgeons on the medical staff seek to remove a surgeon's staff privileges so that there will be less competition for patients, a claim for respondeat superior can be alleged.
   a. True
   b. False

7. Res ipsa loquitur shifts the burden of proof to the defendant.
   a. True
   b. False

8. The Patient Self-Determination Act legalized assisted suicide, for example.
   a. True
   b. False

9. Living wills are advance directives that are to be maintained with the patient's health information according to the U.S. Bill of Rights.
   a. True
   b. False

10. The admissibility of health information varies with states.
    a. True
    b. False

*Additional review questions can be found on the CD-ROM.*

Copyright © 2001 by W.B. Saunders Company. All rights reserved.

# Assignments

## 11-1: REFERENCE GUIDE

### Rationale for Assignment:

*Success and competence are not always due to knowing the answer but to being able to find the resource that can provide the answer. This assignment will give you an opportunity to explore the multitude of resources available to a health information management professional in the legal concepts domain.*

### Directions:

1. Select one topic and one kind of health care facility from the lists below. For example, you could select HIV test information for a neighborhood clinic. Additional topics or types of facilities of interest can be used only with prior instructor approval.
2. Develop a reference guide for the topic with information that applies to that type of health care facility. The reference guide should contain information that would be useful to the Health Information Management Professional working in the identified setting to develop policies, procedures, and training materials on this issue.

    The reference guide must contain:

    A. Table of contents
    B. Introduction including the topic and site for the reference material.
    C. Information from each of the following resources. Material relevant to the topic but not specifically to the setting should be included. Reference material must be included from each type of resource. For each resource:
       i. A copy of the law, article, etc. stating its source in MLA format
       ii. Review of each item in a short summary of the pertinent points relative to the selected topic and setting.
       iii. Resources that must be accessed:
           - Federal laws/regulations, e.g., Conditions of Participation
           - State laws/regulations, e.g., licensing rules
           - Recommendations/practice briefs from HIM professional association
           - Recommendations from the professional health care facility, e.g., American Hospital Association for hospitals
           - Accreditation standards, e.g., National Committee on Quality Assurance for Managed Care Organizations for managed care organizations
           - Professional journals
           - Internet websites
    D. List of publications that would be helpful (books and journals)
    E. List of website addresses—URL and website name
3. The reference guide must be in a format that must be self-explanatory for anyone using it.

| Topics: | Types of Health Care Facilities: |
|---|---|
| Privacy of HIV test results | Chemical dependency—inpatient or outpatient |
| Patient rights | Community mental health center |
| Advanced directives | Home health agency |
| Electronic signatures | Long-term care facility |
| E-mail between patient and provider |     Nursing home |
| Compliance |     Developmentally disabled |
| Ethics | Managed care organization |
| Privacy of genetic testing information | Neighborhood health center/clinic |
| On-line consumer health records | Occupational health clinics |
| Drug testing | Outpatient surgery not connected to a hospital |
| | Physician's office |
| | Rehabilitation facility |

*The above assignment is based on an original concept developed by Mary Teslow, MLS, RHIA. Revised by Ellen B. Jacobs, MEd, RHIA.*

## 11-2: AUTHORIZATION FOR RELEASE OF INFORMATION

Using the principles of forms design from Chapter 3, design a one-page authorization form for release of health information. The form must comply with the requirements of the Federal Regulations on Confidentiality of Alcohol and Drug Abuse Patient Records.

## 11-3: DEVELOPMENT OF A RELEASE OF INFORMATION DATABASE

### Case Study:

One of the responsibilities of the newly hired supervisor in the hospital health information management department is the release of information function. The HIM Director has expressed concern that this area is disorganized and backlogged.

The supervisor reviews the situation and discovers that the easy requests are done first. They are usually sent out within 4 or 5 days. The Correspondence Clerk dislikes the more complicated requests and puts them off, sometimes for weeks. Some requests for information have not been answered for 4 to 5 weeks. In some cases, people who have requested information and not received it have sent second requests or have telephoned him several times before receiving the requested information.

The clerk keeps no records of requests received or responses sent out. He sends out bills to cover copy expenses with the requested information, but he does not monitor whether the bills are paid.

He receives approximately 400 requests a month and currently has a backlog of 225 cases older than 2 weeks of receipt of the request. He understands the confidentiality laws and seems to have no problem regarding sending out information illegally.

The supervisor suspects the reasons he is behind is disorganization, too much talking, and lack of a system to monitor what he does. The supervisor decides to work with him personally on organization skills and keeping to business during work hours. An additional tool that would aid this process is a computer tracking system that could be done on the personal computer he uses for word processing. Because this pc is on a network, the supervisor can access it to determine how well he is doing on a daily basis and to obtain monthly reports related to this activity.

## Assignment:

1. Using the information on database systems from Chapter 4: Data Quality and Technology and information on release of information from Chapter 11: Health Law Concepts and Practices, prepare a matrix (table) using a word processing, spreadsheet or other computer program. In the left column of the matrix, specify the data **FIELDS** to be included in this database. List each field name on a separate row. Be very specific: for example, the patient name would be in two fields, last name and first name/middle initial. Prepare additional columns for **FIELD TYPE, FIELD WIDTH, CODING SCHEME AND EDITS**. Complete the matrix by filling in information for each data field.

2. Part 2-A is for students who have not had instruction on relational database software applications. Refer to Part 2-B for students who have had instruction on using a relational database software program.

    A. Prepare format specifications for the two following reports to be given to the computer programmer. Prepare the format of the reports; provide titles of rows, columns, or sections. Provide enough fictitious data to demonstrate to the programmer how the reports should look.

    i. Release of Information Log. List the data to be included for each patient on whom information was requested and the status of the request..

    ii. Report on the Activities and Work Accomplished by the Correspondence Clerk. This report will go to the supervisor and the department director each month. This report should include information that will be helpful in managing this function, e.g., number of pages copied, number of requests received and sent, dates of requests not answered longer than one week, etc.).

    B. For students who have had instruction in relational database software applications

    i. Using a relational database management program, prepare the main episode/master table as well as other tables.

    ii. Prepare a computer screen form to enter your data.

    iii. Do a "screen dump/print" and print out the tables and entry form(s) you have prepared.

    iv. Enter five cases of fictitious data using your data entry form.

    v. Using database management software, develop:

    a) Release of Information Log itemizing data on each patient on whom requests for information were received, the status and disposition of the request, and the information that was released. This report should include the five cases of fictitious data you entered in Step iv, above. Print a report in which the data are sorted in date order (the date the information was mailed to the requester). Print a second report in alphabetical order by patient last name.

    b) Report on the Activities and Work Accomplished by the Correspondence Clerk. This report will go to the supervisor and the department director each month. This report should include information that will be helpful in managing this function, e.g., number of pages copied, number of requests received and sent, dates of requests not answered longer than one week, etc.). This report should include the five cases of fictitious data you entered in Step iv, above.

## 11-4: RELEASE OF INFORMATION SCENARIOS

## Directions:

*For each scenario, determine the appropriate response.*

## Scenario 1:

A substance abuse program receives a valid authorization to release information to the patient's new therapist, who plans to see that patient for the second time next month. The authorization asks for a copy of the patient's discharge summary. The therapist has just called, and also asked for copies of any discharge summaries on file from any previous care providers or facilities.

## Question:

List all of the information/documents that would be sent to the new therapist in response to this request.

## Scenario 2:

An emergency department physician in a hospital in another city is calling to request information to assist in diagnosing and treating an unconscious patient who is alone. The patient's driver's license reveals that he lives in your town. The physician wants to know whether this patient has been treated at your facility (a general, acute care hospital) and, if so, whether the patient has any significant health problems or allergies. The patient's condition is critical with unknown, multiple injuries from a motor vehicle accident.

## Question:

List the steps needed to respond to this request and to protect the patient's privacy.

## Scenario 3:

Assume the same facts as in Scenario 2, except that review of the patient's record reveals that he is HIV positive. This fact is very important to the Emergency Department staff caring for that patient.

## Question:

How does this alter the response from Situation 2? List the steps to respond to this request.

### Scenario 4:

An adult patient is temporarily unconscious as a result of an accident. The patient's family would like to review the patient's complete medical record.

### Question:

Should the sister, a nurse, be allowed access? Justify your answer.

### Scenario 5:

A physician member of the hospital medical staff asks to see the record from the most recent hospitalization of Joe Smith.

### Question:

What is the first question that should be asked of the doctor?

## 11-5: PROCEDURE FOR FAXING CONFIDENTIAL HEALTH INFORMATION

Using AHIMA guidelines and any applicable state and federal laws, develop a step-by-step procedure to be followed by a health information department employee when faxing confidential health information in response to a valid authorization.

## 11-6: RESPONDING TO A SUBPOENA DUCES TECUM

### Scenario:

The health information management department received a valid subpoena duces tecum by proper service along with the proper witness fee, official seal of the court, and signatures for the medical records of Lee Jackson. Mr. Jackson is the defendant in the case, and the subpoena came from the plaintiff's attorney. The following letter is found on the patient's record.

Health Information Department
Nightingale Memorial Hospital
Nebraska City, NE 99999

To Whom It May Concern:

Please don't release any information from my records to anyone unless I say it is OK. Don't even tell anyone I was a patient there. I could lose my job if you do this. Thank you for your cooperation.

Sincerely,


Lee Jackson

### Assignment:

Explain how to respond to this situation.

## 11-7: INFORMED CONSENT IN HOME HEALTH CARE

### Scenario:

The HIM professional at the StayAtHome Home Health Agency has been asked to respond to the following need:

StayAtHome contracts with a residential behavioral health care facility to provide the medical care when needed. The residents are mainly physically healthy but have behavioral needs, hence living in the residence. The residents have signed a general consent for treatment on admission to the facility. This consent for treatment does not include any services provided by StayAtHome. StayAtHome does have some policies that address this situation, as follows:

### StayAtHome Home Health Agency
### Policies on Obtaining Informed Consent:

#### Who Must Obtain a Patient's Informed Consent for Treatment?

Every health care provider who treats a patient has a legal and ethical duty to obtain the patient's informed consent before commencing treatment. This obligation applies to "practice by referral." Referring physicians often issue generic treatment orders such as "evaluate and treat" and, therefore, practically cannot know what treatment procedures will be performed. The individual provider will know more about the specific treatment modalities than the referring physician and is therefore in a better position to explain proposed treatments and answer patient questions.

#### How Often Must Informed Consent Be Obtained?
A new informed consent must be obtained when:
1. The patient begins treatment with StayAtHome Home Health Agency
2. The original treatment plan is substantially changed
3. A new treatment modality is used

#### How to Tell if a Patient Is Competent to Consent to Treatment
Lack of competency to consent for treatment may result from a patient's unconsciousness, the influence of drugs or intoxicants, mental illness, or other permanent or temporary impairment of reasoning power. The essential determination to be made is whether the patient has sufficient mental ability to understand the situation and make a rational decision as to treatment.

Whenever possible, the provider of services contemplating treatment of a person arguably incompetent should try to obtain "substitute consent" from the person's next of kin in the order prescribed by state law or a court order authorizing treatment. Methods used to obtain the substitute consent and verification of the substitute must be documented in the patient's medical record.

### Problem:

Often the residents seen by StayAtHome's visiting nurses and occupational, physical, and speech therapists are not competent to consent to treatment. No family member/guardian is present at this time of the visit to give informed consent and sign the consent for treatment form. StayAtHome's attorney advised them to create a form that states that the provider (nurses and therapists) obtained verbal consent from the patient's durable power of attorney for health care or legal guardian, etc if the patient was not competent to give consent at the time of treatment. This form should also state that whoever gave the consent will be faxing/mailing the consent form to the agency.

## Assignment:

Respond to this situation as if you are the HIM professional at StayAtHome. The response should include:

1. A memo to the Executive Director of StayAtHome Home Health Agency.
2. A procedure the providers should follow when they encounter this situation.
3. The form(s) to be used when this situation is encountered.

## Evaluation:

Evaluation of this assignment will be based on:

1. The memo, procedure, and forms are clearly and concisely written to reflect the work of an HIM professional.
2. The procedure includes:
    A. Method(s) and criteria for determining if the patient is competent to consent for treatment.
    B. Method and criteria for determining the person who is responsible for authorizing treatment for the patient.
    C. Securing an informed consent for treatment from the responsible party.
    D. Obtaining evidence of the informed consent process for inclusion in the patient's medical record.
3. Consent for treatment forms use language that is understandable to most people.
4. The consent form provides evidence of the informed consent process.
5. References are included.
6. Forms follow the forms design principles.

## 11-8: THOUGHT QUESTIONS

1. Give two examples of acceptable redisclosures of health information.
2. When a health care organization uses a home-based medical transcriptionist, describe one safeguard that should be in place to protect the confidentiality of health information and one that should be in place to protect the security of that health information.
3. List at least two parties, in addition to the HIM professional, who should be involved in developing a health care facility's policy on release of health information to the press. Justify the inclusion of these individuals.
4. Can you ignore a subpoena or a subpoena duces tecum that is clearly defective (some key ingredient is missing)? Explain your answer.
5. Is health information always admissible as evidence in court? Explain your answer.
6. May patients always have access to their own health information? Explain your answer.
7. Which one of the following parties would be an "unauthorized" user of health information? Explain your selection.
    A. The physician consultant asked for a second opinion by the attending physician.
    B. The coder who retrieves the patient record of her new neighbor out of curiosity.
    C. The transcriptionist who suddenly realizes that the report he is typing is about someone he knows.

8. List and briefly explain the four elements of negligence.
9. In Question 8, the four elements of negligence should have been listed in a particular order. Explain the significance of the order of elements.
10. Assume that in a medical malpractice trial alleging that a sponge was left in a surgical site, exactly 50% of the evidence favors the defendant surgeon, and 50% favors the plaintiff. Who is likely to win the case and why?
11. Assume that at a medical malpractice trial alleging postoperative infection, exactly 50% of the evidence favors the plaintiff, and 50% of the evidence favors the defendant physician and hospital. Among the defendant's evidence is some indication that the patient did not comply with postoperative care instructions, including taking antibiotics to fight infection. Who is likely to win the case and why?
12. Assume that an employee of a hospital's HIM department inappropriately released confidential information to a patient's employer. The patient is suing for breach of confidentiality. List all of the parties who could be held liable for this breach, and explain why they are included on the list.

# Review Answers

## PRETEST REVIEW ANSWER KEY

### Directions:

1. Correct your Pretest answers with the answers below by placing a slash through the incorrect question number (Example: 8) with a pen or pencil of a contrasting color.
2. Record the correct answer by placing a square around the letter of the correct answer.
3. Record the total correct on the Initial Performance Grid in Section 4 of this review manual.
4. Calculate your performance rate and also record on the grid.
5. Promptly locate the correct answer for each question missed in the chapter of the textbook.
6. Proceed to the chapter review if your performance rate was 80% or higher; otherwise, return to the chapter for further study.

### Answers to Pretest Review:

1. a
2. b
3. a
4. a
5. a
6. b
7. a
8. a
9. a
10. b

## CHAPTER REVIEW ANSWER KEY

### Directions:

1. Correct your answers with the answers below by placing a slash through the incorrect question number (Example: 8) with a pen or pencil of a contrasting color.
2. Record the correct answer by placing a square around the letter of the correct answer.
3. Record the total correct on the Initial Performance Grid in Section 4 of this review manual.
4. Calculate your performance rate and also record on the grid.
5. Promptly locate the correct answer for each question missed in the chapter of the textbook.
6. Proceed to the next chapter assigned in your study.

### Answers to Chapter Review:

1. a
2. b
3. constitutional
4. a
5. a
6. b
7. a
8. b
9. b
10. a

Copyright © 2001 by W.B. Saunders Company. All rights reserved.

# CHAPTER 12

# Principles of Management

## Review

### PRETEST REVIEW

### Directions:

1. *Read each question carefully before selecting an answer.*
2. *Circle the letter of the correct answer.*
3. *Answer all the questions since there is no penalty for this pretest review.*
4. *Check your answers with the answer key located at the end of this chapter.*

1. Power is a function of a person's position in an organization.
   a. True
   b. False

2. Behavioral decision theory focuses on the decision maker while normative theory focuses on the process.
   a. True
   b. False

3. Planning involves carefully correcting deviations of actual performance from desired performance.
   a. True
   b. False

4. During the stage setting and preparation phase of planning, the organizational mission should be clearly established.
   a. True
   b. False

5. Long-range plans should logically develop from shorter-range plans.
   a. True
   b. False

6. A budget is an intermediate-range plan.
   a. True
   b. False

7. The formal hierarchy in an organization is called the unified command.
   a. True
   b. False

8. Authority is a person's right to require or prohibit certain actions.
   a. True
   b. False

9. Controlling, like planning and organizing, can be accurately thought of as a process involving several steps.

    a. True
    b. False

10. The difference between the planned desired performance and actual performance is the variance.

    a. True
    b. False

# CHAPTER REVIEW

## Directions:

1. *Read each question carefully before selecting an answer.*
2. *Circle the letter of the correct answer.*
3. *Answer all the questions since there is no penalty for this pretest review.*
4. *Check your answers with the answer key located at the end of this chapter.*

1. Span of control states that organizations benefit most when employees use their natural endowments to do what they do best.
   a. True
   b. False

2. Situational management concepts are an important aspect of the contingency theory of management.
   a. True
   b. False

| **Job Title:** | Systems Programmer/Technical Support |
|---|---|
| **Classification:** | Exempt Salaried |
| **Description of Responsibility:** | Accountable for implementation, maintenance, and evaluation of systems software, telecommunications software and support, and coordination of operations. Accountable for all phases of support of data processing systems functions. |

**Typical Tasks:**

1. Develop, plan, implement, and maintain network and data base systems.
2. Evaluate software and hardware changes to enhance and maintain high levels of system performance.
3. Provide technical assistance in areas of problem identification, debugging, and trouble shooting.
4. Provide technical interface among hardware and software vendors, in-house operators, and users.
5. Ensure adequate documentation and training on new system software installations.
6. Generate new projects relating to developing technologies and work improvements.
7. Install and maintain system software, utilities, language processors, access methods, and teleprocessing support.
8. Develop, monitor, maintain, and report on system performance measures.

| **Reporting Relationship:** | Reports to Associate Administrator and Systems and Programming Manager. Coordinative relationship with Projects Manager. |
|---|---|
| **Qualifications:** | B. S. degree in mathematics, computer science, physical sciences, statistics, or accounting. Five years experience in technical data processing and knowledge of data base management, operating system software, data communications, and networking techniques. |

3. Referring to the information in the box on the previous page, what is the name for this management tool?

4. Referring to the information in the box on the previous page, to whom is this employee accountable?

5. Referring to the information in the box on the previous page, which of the six elements will be used in a performance appraisal?

> The Office of Internal Audit provides consultative and educational services in the identification, evaluation, and control of administrative, operational, financial, informational, compliance, and technological risks. We provide these services to distinct administrative units for the benefit of the Audit Committee of the Board of Directors in an objective, ethical, discreet, and professional manner.

6. Referring to the information in the box immediately above, what name is given to this kind of statement?

7. The theory of bureaucracy is most often identified with the Frenchman Henri Fayol.
   a. True
   b. False

8. Frederick Taylor is recognized as the "Father of Scientific Management."
   a. True
   b. False

9. Scientific management is accurately referred to as the functional school of thought.
   a. True
   b. False

10. Situational management emphasizes the importance of basing management actions on universal principles of organization.
    a. True
    b. False

*Additional review questions can be found on the CD-ROM.*

# Assignments

## 12-1: WHAT MAKES A MANAGER?

### Scenario:

It was finally over! The annual employee recognition dinner and awards banquet for University Hospital was history. Now it was time to enjoy the meal and talk to good friends and colleagues. This was the only thing that kept people coming to the ceremony—that and the threat of the CEO to terminate any manager who did not attend and act interested.

At the table where Joan Bell, Director of Nursing, and Judy Reid, Director of Information systems, were sitting, things were especially interesting. Joan had received this year's award for most innovative leader and Judy received the award for highest performing unit. Both were happy and very willing to share their winning philosophy. "Tell me," said Betty Harris, M.D., "what makes a good manager?" "Really, isn't management just common sense?"

Joan took up the challenge first. "If being understanding, flexible, and diplomatic in all dealings with patients, employees, and representatives from other organizations is common sense, I guess you are right. Understanding, flexibility, and diplomacy to all people, in my view, are the secrets of good management."

"Your diplomacy does a disservice to management," Judy protested. "Dr. Harris does us all an injustice by equating management and common sense, and Joan, you don't help very much. Your touchy-feely view of management is what robs us of the respect we should have for doing a very hard and constantly demanding job!"

According to Judy, good managers communicate with employees and let them know what is expected. If they perform, they are rewarded. If they don't perform up to expectations, they get a warning, and if improvements are not forthcoming, they are replaced. Patients should be treated with respect as should their families, but the hospital is a place where people come to get well, not to get pampered. And, as for representatives of other organizations, if the representatives are vendors, "we should, quite simply, stick it to them and get the best deals we can for our hospital. All this diplomacy comes at a cost and vendors perceive it as a weakness!" The fact is, "management is hard work, doing your homework, looking out for our employer, sticking to the rules and policies, and operating efficiently. That, Dr. Harris, is not common sense!"

Bill Baker was recently promoted to supervisor in Judy's unit and he followed the discussion with great interest. He had great respect for Judy and he knew that Joan was recognized throughout the hospital as an outstanding manager. Yet, these two award-winning managers had very different ideas about management. How could they possess such different views of management?

### Questions:

1. Let's begin with Bill's question. How could two outstanding managers possess such different views of management?
2. Can these two views be reconciled? Is it possible both managers could be right? Why or why not?
3. What would you say to Bill who is attempting to develop his own management philosophy? Would you recommend the ideas of Judy or Joan? Explain your advice to Bill.

Copyright © 2001 by W.B. Saunders Company. All rights reserved.

## 12-2: ALLEN SIMPSON'S LEADERSHIP PLAN

### Scenario:

Allen Simpson is director of health information systems at Lakeview Health Services. He is responsible for supervising a group of information systems professionals. Most of the employees in his unit are young, recent college graduates, and several have graduate degrees.

Allen has been a manager for more than 20 years and as such has directly supervised a couple of generations of health professionals. When he first accepted a management position, he believed that most professional employees wanted autonomy—to be left alone to do their jobs with a minimum of supervision. Several actually told him not to bother them with administrative details. "Just give us the goals and get out of the way" was a frequent comment from his attempts to get input from employees. As a result, Allen developed an autocratic leadership style. According to him, "If people don't want to participate, I can't force them. I will provide goals and assume everyone knows what to do. If they don't, I am always available." No one objected to the style, and his employees have always performed very well.

In the late 1980s, Allen began to detect some changes. Several of his best employees suggested that they had some ideas for improving operations and thought he might want to listen to them. He was uncomfortable with the approach and always worried that people were really thinking, "What does Allen get paid for if he is always asking for my ideas?" Over time, however, he became more comfortable with the participative approach and has done a very good job of involving people in decision making.

Recently, Allen has sensed another change among his younger employees. "They seem more like the ones I supervised when I first became a manager." They are not so anxious to provide their input and suggestions. In fact, according to Allen, "They are very myopic and seem to relate only to their jobs rather than looking at the big picture." Once again, he has been forced to alter his style of management and leadership. At team meetings, most of the younger employees seem bored. Many do not arrive until well after the meeting has started and then excuse their tardiness with comments like "I was in the middle of something really important and just could not break away."

Simpson was confused but not frustrated. He had changed his style from autocratic to participative before and saw no reason why he could not change from participative to autocratic. If people did not want to be involved, he could make decisions without them!

### Questions:

1. What do you think about Allen Simpson's dilemma? Should he continue to change his style based on his perceptions of employee preferences?
2. How can Allen deal with each new generation of employees without the necessity of radically altering his leadership style?
3. Do you think Simpson faces a problem unique to professional employees or is it representative of employees in general?

## 12-3: ASSESSING AN ORGANIZATION

### Directions:

*Answer the following for either your current or past employer or a professional practice site. Utilize an organization chart if available.*

1. Mission, Vision, and Values
    A. What is the organization's mission?
    B. Where did you first hear about the organizational mission?
    C. Do your colleagues generally understand the mission?
    D. How is the mission communicated throughout the organization?
    E. What about the vision of the organization; do they know where they are going and how you relate to the organization's future?
    F. Does anyone talk about the vision and use it to excite employees about their future? If so, who is the "keeper of the vision"?
    G. What are the fundamental values of this organization (what does the organization stand for)?
2. Structure
    A. How is the organization structured?
    B. How would you describe the departmentalization philosophy underlying the organization—functional, geographic, etc.?
    C. Does the structure reflect the strategy, mission, vision, etc. of the organization? Explain your response.
3. Objectives and Goals
    A. Do you have clearly understood goals or objectives for your job?
    B. Do your individual goals and objectives relate to the organizational mission and vision? If so, how? If not, how would you suggest improving the relationship between organizational mission, group, and individual goals?

## 12-4: MEDICAL ASSOCIATES, INC.

### Case Study:

Elizabeth Copuis began working for the Medical Associates, Inc. while she majored in journalism at Fairmont College. Fairmont was her hometown so it was convenient for her to work in the afternoon and take classes in the morning and evening. Throughout the three years of part-time work, she held a variety of positions including clerk typist, receptionist, and computer operator.

Her work was so satisfactory that she was offered a full-time job as supervisor in one of the information system areas upon her graduation from Fairmont. She accepted the job and within three months was promoted to computer operations supervisor. As computer operations supervisor, she missed some of the hands-on tasks but was convinced she could improve turnover by almost 100 percent. She devised and implemented a new incentive program to encourage aggressive employee involvement in decision making. Weekly, she met withall employees under her supervision, although it was time consuming, to discuss their problems, concerns, and performance.

The success of Elizabeth soon caught the attention of top management. Several key executives encouraged her to apply for the M.B.A. program at a well-known Eastern university. She was accepted and the company granted her a two-year educational leave of absence with pay.

Upon return to Medical Associates with her graduate training, Elizabeth was promoted to director of marketing, a key person on the middle management team. In this position, she was responsible for coordinating several departments including marketing and management information systems. As director of marketing, she spent much of her time ensuring that all areas of marketing and management information systems were closely coordinated. This frequently involved resolving conflicts that developed between the two groups. She was especially effective, however, in developing project teams or task forces, as she liked to call them, to expose and solve pressing marketing problems.

Last week Elizabeth Copuis was promoted to executive vice president of operations. In this job, she is one of the top four officers of the company and is directly involved in executive decision making. One of her primary duties is to forecast future trends and developments in the strategies for marketing Medical Associates services and for introducing new ones. She is also expected to "interface" with trade associations and ensure that the legislative interests of Medical Associates are made known to influential politicians.

### Questions:

1. Briefly explain how Elizabeth Copuis' career has developed according to the progressive responsibility path.
2. Develop one alternative way that her career could have evolved after she returned with her M.B.A.

## 12-5: SOUTH LAND MANAGED CARE

### Case Study:

The South Land Managed Care is a subsidiary of Ecosystems International. Throughout its history, South Land Managed Care has relied on Ecosystems International to furnish it with sufficient computer processing time on the home office computer system. In recent years, however, the work has become too demanding and time consuming to be absorbed on the home office computer system. Therefore, South Land leased its own computer hardware from a local computer sales and service company. South Land also hired a director of computer services with a substantial amount of experience in the home office operation.

During the first four months on the job, Mr. Amos, the director, was occupied with planning and getting the new system on-line. Then the trouble began. First, the heads of the various service departments were told the manner in which work had to be submitted if it was to be processed by the computer. Mr. Amos also sold corporate management on the idea that the service departments should be charged with the expense of the computer operations according to a complex formula that only Mr. Amos understood, and he was not willing to carefully explain it to anyone. Even the president could not understand exactly what was happening.

The final act was committed when Mr. Amos sent all department heads a memorandum that asked for the type of reports and data they desired and that would help them to do their jobs better. After looking over the list, Mr. Amos summarized a series of reports that he would supply all departments. Most of the department heads agreed that Mr. Amos's list revealed little relationship to the items they submitted.

One by one the department heads began to appear in the office of the president. The question was: "Who is running this place and isn't the function of the computer department to support service delivery to our members?" Eventually, the problem became so widespread that no one could deny its existence. The president must now make a response to the service delivery departments at the next staff meeting. Some of the issues he is concerned with are:

### Questions:

1. Exactly what is the relationship of service delivery to computer services?
2. How can the problem be resolved without returning to the previous problems of not having adequate computer services?
3. Clearly explain the proper role of a line (service delivery) and a staff (support) unit to the president. How would you organize the computer function at South Land Managed Care?
4. Suggest a way the president can resolve the dilemma of supporting the service units while not "selling out" the computer function.

## 12-6: MEDICAL LABORATORY ENTERPRISES

### Case Study:

Meredith Goddard is an extremely unique individual. She received a B.S. degree in biological sciences from a well-known technical university and a Ph.D. in microbiology from one of the best science departments in the nation. In addition to this, she is a certified medical technologist and worked for several years for a major aerospace corporation as a researcher studying the effects of space travel on bacteria. She was even selected as a possible space scientist and was scheduled to participate in one of NASA's manned space flight programs.

Now, however, she is an executive with Medical Laboratory Enterprises, a corporation that does specialized subcontracting work for a number of medical research centers. When she came to work for Medical Laboratory Enterprises, she was amazed to see the inability of the firm to deal with problems that were temporary in nature. In fact, the company hired her in her present position primarily to redesign the existing organizational structure.

According to Jim Sabbs, vice president for organization development, the major problem with the existing structure is the difficulty the company experiences in dealing with "one-time problems" that constantly occur but are always different than before. For example, Medical Enterprises once obtained the contract from NASA to build the heating cores for the specimen boxes on an unmanned lunar probe mission. The job was technically challenging and required many diverse specialists. None of the specialists were assigned to the same department, and a great deal of conflict developed in acquiring the necessary talent to do the job the corporation had promised to do.

Dr. Goddard suggested that some type of project organization would be best suited for the type of problems faced by Medical Laboratory Enterprises. In a report submitted to the president, she outlined the following reasons she felt consideration should be given to establishing a project structure.

1. The formulation of a project structure would provide a central focal point for the work of the various units and allow for a more centralized cost control.
2. A project structure would make the mobilization of required specialists under a single director relatively simple.
3. A project structure would allow for increased participation in decision making by technical personnel and probably increase morale.
4. The increased participation would also be likely to stimulate creativity and aid in decision making.
4. Finally, the implementation of a project structure would broaden the views of technical personnel when they were forced to work closely with other types of specialists.

The president reviewed the report and was basically pleased. However, he too had spent time in medical laboratories and was not sure he was as impressed with the project structure as was Dr. Goddard. He was in the process of formulating his reply.

### Questions:

1. Help the president formulate his idea by listing some of the potential dangers of the project structure.
2. What cautions would you suggest Dr. Goddard think of before recommending the project structure without excessive enthusiasm?
3. In general, do you agree or disagree with Dr. Goddard's recommendation? Please explain your response.

## 12-7: VALLEY BEHAVIORAL HEALTH HOSPITAL

### Case Study:

Dr. Sharon Bock is the Director of the Valley Behavioral Health Hospital. Valley is a comprehensive care facility equipped for the treatment of all types of behavioral health illness. Last year Dr. Bock began to investigate alternatives for the care and treatment of mildly ill patients.

One of the primary difficulties involved in treatment of this type of patient is that not only must medical problems be considered but also a plan must be developed for deinstitutionalizing the individuals. The latter problem is, in many cases, more serious than the former. The former problem is medical whereas the latter is medical, psychological, social, and so on.

To prepare patients for their reentry into noninstitutionalized life, many specialists must be involved with the patient and his or her family.

Because of this multidisciplinary necessity, Dr. Bock decided to experiment with an organizational alternative that could more effectively satisfy patient needs. To develop this alternative, Dr. Bock asked the staff for suggestions and offered a series of training seminars on modern developments in the care and treatment of behavioral illness. The main thrust of the "new philosophy" was to impress on the staff the importance of carefully working with all dimensions of the patient's needs.

The consensus in all the participation sessions was that a multidisciplinary team must be formulated to work with the patient. This team would require the services of a physician, nurse, psychologist, social worker, and occupational therapist. An experimental team, or unit as Dr. Bock called it, was created and allowed a great deal of flexibility and freedom.

Everything seemed to go well within the unit. The team members were dedicated to the concept of deinstitutionalization, and the patients responded well. The real problem developed with respect to the other organizational units.

Complaints were frequently heard about the unusual freedom given to the experimental unit. Even some patients who were not selected to participate had verbally abused the patients in the unit. One patient had become so upset by the abuse that his condition had significantly declined. Dr. Hailey, the unit psychologist, also had a confrontation with a staff psychologist. Dr. Bock could no longer deny that problems existed in the experimental unit. This was very hard for her to understand. She had tried very hard to implement an innovative change in the proper way.

### Questions:

1. What do you think has caused the problem in the experimental unit?
2. How could the problem have been approached differently? What would you do now?

# Review Answers

## PRETEST REVIEW ANSWER KEY

### Directions:

1. Correct your Pretest answers with the answers below by placing a slash through the incorrect question number (Example: 8) with a pen or pencil of a contrasting color.
2. Record the correct answer by placing a square around the letter of the correct answer.
3. Record the total correct on the Initial Performance Grid in Section 4 of this review manual.
4. Calculate your performance rate and also record on the grid.
5. Promptly locate the correct answer for each question missed in the chapter of the textbook.
6. Proceed to the chapter review if your performance rate was 80% or higher; otherwise, return to the chapter for further study.

### Answers to Pretest Review:

| | | | | |
|---|---|---|---|---|
| 1. | a | | 6. | b |
| 2. | a | | 7. | b |
| 3. | b | | 8. | a |
| 4. | a | | 9. | a |
| 5. | b | | 10. | a |

## CHAPTER REVIEW ANSWER KEY

### Directions:

1. Correct your answers with the answers below by placing a slash through the incorrect question number (Example: 8) with a pen or pencil of a contrasting color.
2. Record the correct answer by placing a square around the letter of the correct answer.
3. Record the total correct on the Initial Performance Grid in Section 4 of this review manual.
4. Calculate your performance rate and also record on the grid.
5. Promptly locate the correct answer for each question missed in the chapter of the textbook.
6. Proceed to the next chapter assigned in your study.

### Answers to Chapter Review:

| | | | | |
|---|---|---|---|---|
| 1. | b | | 6. | mission statement |
| 2. | a | | 7. | b |
| 3. | job description | | 8. | a |
| 4. | Associate Administrator & Systems and Programming Manager | | 9. | b |
| 5. | typical tasks | | 10. | b |

# CHAPTER 13

# OPERATIONAL MANAGEMENT

## Review

### PRETEST REVIEW

### Directions:

1. *Read each question carefully before selecting an answer.*
2. *Circle the letter of the correct answer.*
3. *Answer all the questions since there is no penalty for this pretest review.*
4. *Check your answers with the answer key located at the end of this chapter.*

1. Which document indicates how much time employees in a department spend on various activities?

   a. organization chart
   b. flowchart
   c. flow process chart
   d. work distribution chart

2. A step on a flow process chart that states "arranges sheets in alphabetical order" would be characterized as a(an):

   a. operation
   b. verification
   c. delay
   d. transportation

3. When completing a work distribution chart, the first task is usually to:

   a. determine the job position for each employee in the department
   b. have each employee complete a list of his or her daily activities/duties

   c. have each supervisor complete a list of the daily activities/duties of his or her subordinates
   d. have the department director complete a list of the daily activities/duties of each employee

4. Which is a visual tool that combines the relationship of work planned, work completed, and time is called a:

   a. work distribution chart
   b. flow process chart
   c. PERT network
   d. Gantt chart

5. In work sampling, how should the observation times of the worker's tasks be scheduled?

   a. sequentially
   b. randomly
   c. periodically
   d. continuously

6. In order for a manager to encourage the acceptance of standards in a department, she/he should:
   a. suspend employees who consistently do not meet the standards
   b. cut the wages of employees who consistently do not meet the standards
   c. involve the employees in the development of the standards
   d. involve the employees in deciding whether the standards should be applied in any particular case

7. The width of a main aisle in most office areas should be about:
   a. 15 feet
   b. 10 feet
   c. 5 feet
   d. 3 feet

8. When the department director compares actual departmental performance against pre-established standards, which of the following management principles is being utilized?
   a. planning
   b. organizing
   c. controlling
   d. actuating

9. Color has a significant influence upon the lighting of an office.
   a. True
   b. False

10. The spacing of file cabinets depends upon the frequency of their use and upon the type of cabinet.
    a. True
    b. False

# CHAPTER REVIEW

## Directions:

*1. Read each question carefully before selecting an answer.*
*2. Circle the letter of the correct answer.*
*3. Answer all the questions since there is no penalty for this pretest review.*
*4. Check your answers with the answer key located at the end of this chapter.*

1. A Gantt chart would be useful in which of the following activities?
   a. phasing
   b. cycling
   c. scheduling
   d. activating

2. When constructing a PERT network, time is generally related to:
   a. events
   b. activities
   c. dummy activities
   d. merge events

3. A work distribution chart:
   a. shows how much work each employee produces daily
   b. accounts for every minute of time that an employee spends on the job
   c. distributes work equally among employees in a section or department
   d. shows the type of work performed and the time spent on each task by each employee

4. A step on a flow process chart that indicates "brought to the inactive file" would be characterized as a (an):
   a. operation
   b. transportation
   c. delay
   d. verification

5. The goal of work simplification is:
   a. smooth flow of work
   b. elimination of waste
   c. control of procedures
   d. employee participation

6. It has been determined that it takes .356 of an hour on average to assemble and analyze one patient record for deficiencies, and it has been projected that there will be 14,520 discharges in the coming year. How many personnel hours will be needed to assemble and analyze this volume of charts?
   a. 3050
   b. 3500
   c. 5169
   d. 5196

7. What is the first question that a work simplification analyst should ask?
   a. When is it done and why?
   b. How many personnel use it and why?
   c. What is being done and why?
   d. Who does it and why?

8. You are given four proposals for an enhanced layout of the clerical area of your department. In reviewing the proposals, you discover that each presents a different proposed amount of space for the clerks. You then decide that you will follow the accepted space guidelines for clerical workers and make a final decision from the proposals presented. Which of the following will you accept:
   a. 5' x 10' per clerical worker
   b. 5' x 12' per clerical worker
   c. 5' x 15' per clerical worker
   d. 10' x 10' per clerical worker

Copyright © 2001 by W.B. Saunders Company. All rights reserved.

9. In order to file the greatest number of hard copy medical records in the least amount of space, which of the following types of equipment would you use?

    a. drawer files
    b. movable aisle files
    c. open shelf files
    d. lateral file cabinets

10. Task/ambient lighting directs light to a specific area (that is, where the worker needs light the most) instead of indiscriminately throughout the office.

    a. True
    b. False

*Additional review questions can be found on the CD-ROM.*

# Assignments

## 13-1: WORK DISTRIBUTION CHART

### Assignment:

Develop a work distribution chart for the Release of Information/Correspondence Work Unit of a Health Information Department using the following task lists for the:

- Supervisor
- Receptionist
- Subpoena Clerk
- Correspondence Clerk

1. Determine the activity categories to be used on the Work Distribution Chart based on the tasks listed for the individual employee. List the activities in order of importance to the overall goals of the work unit. Be sure each task from the task lists can be grouped into one activity category. Tasks should not be included in more than one category.

2. Using the task lists, the activity categories, and following worksheet, develop a work distribution chart for the Release of Information/Correspondence area of the Health Information Department. All activities for all staff should be included in the chart. The total hours from each staff member's activity list should equal the total hours on the work distribution chart.

3. Using the questions listed in Chapter 13 in the book, analyze the work distribution chart.

4. Develop a memo to the Director of the Health Information Department with a description of the findings and recommendations for changes in the work unit.

5. Create a new work distribution chart that shows your recommended changes.

## Task Lists

*Department/Area: Release of Information/Correspondence*
*Date Compiled: 02/01/200X–02/05/200X*

*Job Title: Receptionist*

| Task Number | Activities | Hours Per Week |
|---|---|---|
| 1. | Answers phone | 12 |
| 2. | Greets visitors to department | 6 |
| 3. | Picks up mail from the mailroom | 5 |
| 4. | Assists in other departmental functions | 9 |
| 5. | Keeps Hospital Directory current | 1 |
| 6. | Miscellaneous (breaks, lunch) | 7 |

*Job Title: Subpoena Clerk*

| Task Number | Activities | Hours Per Week |
|---|---|---|
| 1. | Receives subpoena from supervisor | 2 |
| 2. | Processes requests by subpoena | 5 |
| 3. | Pulls records and makes copies to respond to subpoenas | 10 |
| 4. | Prepares copies for mail responses to subpoenas | 9 |
| 5. | Processes mail requests for information | 3 |
| 6. | Verifies information from attorneys | 4 |
| 7. | Miscellaneous (breaks, lunch) | 7 |

## Task Lists

*Department/Area: Release of Information/Correspondence*
*Date Compiled: 02/01/2000 - 02/05/2000*

*Job Title: Supervisor*

| Task Number | Activities | Hours Per Week |
|---|---|---|
| 1. | Supervisory duties | 15 |
| 2. | Handles problems with attorneys | 5 |
| 3. | Accepts subpoenas | 3 |
| 4. | Computes release of information statistics | 4 |
| 5. | Court appearances | 1 |
| 6. | Meetings | 5 |
| 7. | Miscellaneous (breaks lunch) | 7 |

*Job Title: Correspondence Clerk*

| Task Number | Activities | Hours Per Week |
|---|---|---|
| 1. | Processes mail requests for information | 5 |
| 2. | Locates and copies record | 8 |
| 3. | Documents responses | 5 |
| 4. | Receives requests for faxing of records | 4 |
| 5. | Processes requests for faxed information | 9 |
| 6. | Verifies information from attorneys | 3 |
| 7. | Miscellaneous (lunch, breaks) | 6 |

# Work Distribution Chart

Section: Release of Information/Correspondence
Date Compiled: _____
Department: Health Information Management
Work Group: _____

| Tasks | Supervisor | Hrs | Subpoena Clerk | Hrs | Correspondence Clerk | Hrs | Receptionist | Hrs | Total Hrs |
|---|---|---|---|---|---|---|---|---|---|
|  |  |  |  |  |  |  |  |  |  |
|  |  |  |  |  |  |  |  |  |  |
|  |  |  |  |  |  |  |  |  |  |
|  |  |  |  |  |  |  |  |  |  |
|  |  |  |  |  |  |  |  |  |  |
|  |  |  |  |  |  |  |  |  |  |
|  |  |  |  |  |  |  |  |  |  |
|  |  |  |  |  |  |  |  |  |  |
| Total |  |  |  |  |  |  |  |  |  |

## 13-2: TRANSCRIPTION PRODUCTIVITY STUDY

The director of the Health Information Management Department at Anywhere Regional Medical Center (a 500-bed facility) wants to:

- Analyze the productivity of the transcription area.
- Determine the number of personnel needed for this function during the next budget period.

## Questions:

Use the information provided below to answer the following questions:

1. Total lines typed per **month** by all three transcriptionists
2. Total lines typed per **year** by all three transcriptionists
3. **Average** number of lines typed per year per transcriptionist
4. Total lines per year predicted for next budget year
5. How many additional transcriptionists in F.T.E. (round to one decimal point) will be needed to complete the work for the next budget period?

### Transcription Statistics

Average Typed Lines per Page: 45

Average Typed Lines per Report:

| Reports | Average Lines per Report | Annual Figures |
| --- | --- | --- |
| History & Physical | 90 | (2 pages) |
| Discharge Summary | 45 | (1 page) |
| Consultation Report | 112.5 | (2.5 pages) |
| Operative Report | 112.5 | (2.5 pages) |

### Anywhere Medical Center Statistics for the Next Budget Period

| | |
| --- | --- |
| Admissions/discharges | 56,000 |
| Consultations | 45% of all admissions |
| Surgical procedure(s) performed | 75% of all admissions |

## Monthly Transcription Logs

Name: _Susan_

| Transcribed Reports | Week 1 | Week 2 | Week 3 | Week 4 | Total |
|---|---|---|---|---|---|
| History & Physical | 30,200 | 31,350 | 31,300 | 31,405 | |
| Discharge Summary | 16,175 | 15,975 | 15,910 | 15,950 | |
| Consultation Report | 18,750 | 18,925 | 18,837 | 18,942 | |
| Operative Report | 31,600 | 31,325 | 31,570 | 31,495 | |
| Total | | | | | |

Name: _Mary_

| Transcribed Reports | Week 1 | Week 2 | Week 3 | Week 4 | Total |
|---|---|---|---|---|---|
| History & Physical | 30,400 | 31,425 | 31,050 | 30,850 | |
| Discharge Summary | 16,480 | 16,250 | 16,350 | 16,410 | |
| Consultation Report | 18,525 | 18,450 | 18,628 | 18,480 | |
| Operative Report | 31,575 | 31,600 | 31,492 | 31,523 | |
| Total | | | | | |

Name: _Diane_

| Transcribed Reports | Week 1 | Week 2 | Week 3 | Week 4 | Total |
|---|---|---|---|---|---|
| History & Physical | 30,600 | 31,275 | 30,850 | 30,735 | |
| Discharge Summary | 16,320 | 16,125 | 16,253 | 16,305 | |
| Consultation Report | 18,975 | 18,750 | 18,864 | 18,955 | |
| Operative Report | 31,250 | 31,400 | 31,383 | 31,469 | |
| Total | | | | | |

## 13-3: GROUP EXERCISE: CONSTRUCTING A FLOW PROCESS CHART

## Assignment:

1. In groups of three, complete the following flow process chart for the analysis/incomplete chart process by selecting the symbol that best describes each step. Count the number of each of the symbols used and enter the totals in the summary box.
2. Analyze the existing process to see what steps can be eliminated, combined, and resequenced to make it more efficient.
3. From the above analysis, develop a revised process and enter each step in the Proposed Method column of the flow process chart. Select the symbol that best describes each step. Count the number of each symbol used and enter the totals in the summary box.
4. Compute the difference in the number of symbols used in the present and the proposed processes.
5. In a narrative, summarize the changes made to the process and describe how the process will be improved.

214 ■ Study Guide to Accompany *Health Information: Management of a Strategic Resource*

Job _____  Department _____
Charted by _____  Date _____

|  | Present | Proposed | Difference |
|---|---|---|---|
| ○ No. of Operations |  |  |  |
| ⇧ No. of Transportations |  |  |  |
| □ No. of Inspections |  |  |  |
| ◗ No. of Delays |  |  |  |
| ▶ No. of Storages |  |  |  |
| Distance Traveled |  |  |  |
| Minutes Delayed |  |  |  |

| Present Method | Operation | Transportation | Inspection | Delay | Storage | Distance (ft) | Time (min) | Proposed Method | Operation | Transportation | Inspection | Delay | Storage | Distance (ft) | Time (min) |
|---|---|---|---|---|---|---|---|---|---|---|---|---|---|---|---|
| Upon discharge of patient, nursing personnel bring charts to PBX operator | ○ | ⇧ | □ | ◗ | ▶ |  |  |  | ○ | ⇧ | □ | ◗ | ▶ |  |  |
| Operator brings charts to the health information department at 8:00 AM | ○ | ⇧ | □ | ◗ | ▶ |  |  |  | ○ | ⇧ | □ | ◗ | ▶ |  |  |
| Charts waits for tumor registrar review | ○ | ⇧ | □ | ◗ | ▶ |  |  |  | ○ | ⇧ | □ | ◗ | ▶ |  |  |
| Tumor registrar reviews charts | ○ | ⇧ | □ | ◗ | ▶ |  |  |  | ○ | ⇧ | □ | ◗ | ▶ |  |  |
| The discharge clerks pick up charts from front desk after 10:00 AM | ○ | ⇧ | □ | ◗ | ▶ |  |  |  | ○ | ⇧ | □ | ◗ | ▶ |  |  |
| Discharge analysis is done | ○ | ⇧ | □ | ◗ | ▶ |  |  |  | ○ | ⇧ | □ | ◗ | ▶ |  |  |
| Discharge clerks pass charts to the coding clerks | ○ | ⇧ | □ | ◗ | ▶ |  |  |  | ○ | ⇧ | □ | ◗ | ▶ |  |  |

*Continued.*

Copyright © 2001 by W.B. Saunders Company. All rights reserved.

*Continued from previous page.*

| Present Method | Operation | Transportation | Inspection | Delay | Storage | Distance (ft) | Time (min) | Proposed Method | Operation | Transportation | Inspection | Delay | Storage | Distance (ft) | Time (min) |
|---|---|---|---|---|---|---|---|---|---|---|---|---|---|---|---|
| Diagnoses and procedures are coded | ○ | ⇧ | □ | ● | ▶ | | | | ○ | ⇧ | □ | ● | ▶ | | |
| Charts go to discharge clerks | ○ | ⇧ | □ | ● | ▶ | | | | ○ | ⇧ | □ | ● | ▶ | | |
| Clerks attach late reports | ○ | ⇧ | □ | ● | ▶ | | | | ○ | ⇧ | □ | ● | ▶ | | |
| Tumor registrar compiles registry list | ○ | ⇧ | □ | ● | ▶ | | | | ○ | ⇧ | □ | ● | ▶ | | |
| Charts go to incomplete file room | ○ | ⇧ | □ | ● | ▶ | | | | ○ | ⇧ | □ | ● | ▶ | | |
| After physician review, the charts go back to discharge desk | ○ | ⇧ | □ | ● | ▶ | | | | ○ | ⇧ | □ | ● | ▶ | | |
| Charts are checked again | ○ | ⇧ | □ | ● | ▶ | | | | ○ | ⇧ | □ | ● | ▶ | | |
| Charts go back to incomplete file room | ○ | ⇧ | □ | ● | ▶ | | | | ○ | ⇧ | □ | ● | ▶ | | |
| Chart deficiencies are updated in computer | ○ | ⇧ | □ | ● | ▶ | | | | ○ | ⇧ | □ | ● | ▶ | | |
| Completed charts go to coding clerk for final check | ○ | ⇧ | □ | ● | ▶ | | | | ○ | ⇧ | □ | ● | ▶ | | |
| Charts are filed in permanent file | ○ | ⇧ | □ | ● | ▶ | | | | ○ | ⇧ | □ | ● | ▶ | | |

Copyright © 2001 by W.B. Saunders Company. All rights reserved.

## 13-4: PROFESSIONAL PRACTICE: SYSTEMS FLOWCHARTS

### Assignment:

1. Create a systems flowchart of the coding process in a health care facility. Develop separate flowcharts for each of the various types of patient, e.g., inpatient, outpatient, mental health, Medicare, or commercial insured, if they are processed differently.
2. The flowchart should trace the flow of data from the patient encounter to the generation of the bill (electronic or paper). Include in the flow of information:
   - the various operations that occur within the system
   - the files that are accessed
   - the reports produced
   - the applications programs that are required to operate the system
3. Develop additional charts to show how the flow of information differs for:
   - an inpatient versus an outpatient
   - various third-party payers, e.g., Medicare versus Blue Cross

## 13-5: PROFESSIONAL PRACTICE: OPERATIONS/PROCEDURE FLOWCHART

### Assignment:

1. Obtain information about the procedure used to respond to requests for information from the patient record by either reviewing the written procedure or interviewing a Correspondence/Release of Information Clerk.
2. Draw an operations/procedure flowchart illustrating the process followed to release medical information. If available, utilize computer software to create the chart. Limit the chart to the processes that occur within the Health Information Management Department. Include in the chart the sequence of activities and decision points that are encountered in carrying out this function.
3. Evaluate the process in a narrative. Include in the narrative suggestions for making the process more efficient and effective. Justify the recommendations.
4. Draw an operations/procedure flowchart that shows the revised process.

## 13-6: PROFESSIONAL PRACTICE: MOVEMENT DIAGRAM

### Assignment:

1. Illustrate the major pieces of equipment, furniture, and functions on a physical layout of a health information management department. The department may be one you recently visited in a professional practice, a tour, or where you work.
2. Draw a movement diagram on the physical layout showing the flow of the patient record from receipt in the department to permanent file.
3. In a narrative, evaluate the flow of the record identifying bottlenecks and backtracking. Include in the narrative suggestions and justifications for improvements in the work flow. Describe how computerization of the patient record will affect this work flow.
4. Illustrate the recommended changes on a second movement diagram.

## 13-7: GROUP EXERCISE: DECISION MATRIX

### Case Study:

The transcription section of the Health Information Management Department consists of 13 transcriptions that work the following shifts:

| Number of Employees | Days Worked | Shifts |
| --- | --- | --- |
| 7 | Monday–Friday | 7 AM to 3:30 PM |
| 4 | Monday–Friday | 3 PM to 11:30 PM |
| 2 | Monday–Friday | 11 PM to 7:30 AM |

Three transcriptionists, one from day shift and two from evening shift, have requested to work at home via telecommuting.

### Assignment:

1. Form groups of three. Each person in the group will represent one of the following:
   - Chief Financial Officer (The HIM Director's boss)
   - The Director of the Health Information Management Department
   - Transcription Supervisor
2. As a group, develop a decision matrix to determine and evaluate the alternatives to this request. Include in the elements to be considered: cost, feasibility, desirability, acceptance, effect on productivity, and effect on quality.
3. Summarize each alternative and arrive at a consensus.

## 13-8: GROUP EXERCISE: PROJECT MANAGEMENT

### Case Study:
Two hospitals have merged and the master patient indices of both facilities need to be combined.

### Assignment:
1. Working in a group, develop a Project Plan for the merging of the master patient indices for the two hospitals. Select one member of the group to be project leader. Assign the other members to have various areas of expertise.
2. Formulate a problem definition for this project. It must include:
   - Problem statement
   - Goal
   - Objects
   - Resources
3. Formulate a project plan that includes:
   - Project activities
   - Time
   - Cost
   - Activity sequence
   - Critical activities
   - Project proposal

*Note: You may need to make assumptions to develop this plan. Recognize and document the assumptions you made.*

## 13-9: PERT EXERCISE

### Assignment:

1. Utilizing the following data, draw a PERT chart.
2. Determine the critical path and state how long (in days) the critical path will take.

### Case Study:

*The following data apply to a health information management project in a 500-bed hospital.*

| Activity | Expected Time (Days) | Activity | Expected Time (Days) |
|---|---|---|---|
| A-B | 6 | I-L | 5 |
| A-C | 2 | I-K | 1 |
| B-E | 8 | J-L | 2 |
| C-J | 11 | J-M | 2 |
| E-F | 10 | K-O | 6 |
| E-G | 3 | L-N | 7 |
| G-J | 1 | M-N | 8 |
| F-I | 3 | N-O | 6 |

## 13-10: PERT NETWORK

### Case Study:

The Assistant Director has been given the challenge of being a Project Manager for the installation of a computerized record deficiency system in a 300-bed inpatient hospital.

### Assignment:

1. Identify the various components of the project and the estimated completion time of each component.
2. Design a PERT network that illustrates the completion of this project.
3. Identify the critical path and the length of time needed to complete the project.

## 13-11: GANTT CHART

### Case Study:

A large (800-bed) acute care tertiary hospital has paper patient records from 1960 to 2000 stored in the basement of an adjacent warehouse. During this period, there were approximately 10,000 discharges per year. The administration has approved the proposal to convert these records to optical disk.

### Assignment:

Prepare a Gantt chart for this project. Include time units, responsible individuals, and the project work elements.

*Note: Believe it or not, the real hospital has records dating back to 1932!*

## 13-12: WRITING A PROCEDURE

## Assignment:

1. Using one of the methods for writing procedures (narrative, outline, or play script), develop a procedure for the receipt and processing of medical records of discharged patients.
2. The following activities must be completed in order to properly process the medical records of discharged patients:
   - Medical records of discharged patients are retrieved from the patient care units on a daily basis during the 11:00 PM–7:00 AM shift. (health information courier)
   - The records are sorted by discharge date. (analysis clerk)
   - Partial records (records that are not complete and that have other parts of the record filed elsewhere) have to be bound by rubber bands or paper clips. (analysis clerk)
   - The computer has to be queried to see where the corresponding record is for all partial records. In-house partials are placed in premade folders on the "in-house" shelf. For all other partials, the corresponding record should be located and the partial placed inside it. If the record cannot be located, the partial is placed in terminal digit order on the "Partial" shelf. The location of the record in the computer system should be changed to "Recompile." (analysis clerk)
   - Fetal monitor strips have to be removed from the records and placed in labeled envelopes. The patient's name, hospital number, and the date have to be recorded on the envelope. (analysis clerk)
   - These envelopes are then taken to "Permanent File." (file clerk)
   - The coding section has discharge lists that are checked to make sure that there is a chart for each patient. Somehow the patient's name is marked or highlighted to show that a chart was received. After all of the charts are checked, the lists are returned to the coding staff. (analysis clerk)
   - Each record of a discharged patient is placed in a premade folder. A bar code label is made for the patient's name and medical record number and placed on the bottom of the folder. The patient's name and medical record number are also handwritten on the folder. (analysis clerk)
   - The location of each of the discharge records (incomplete charts, coding, etc.) is input into the computer. (analysis clerk)
   - The medical record is sent to the appropriate location for coding, completion by physicians, or filing. (incomplete charts clerk)

## 13-13: OFFICE LAYOUT AND DESIGN PROJECT

### Case Study:

Anywhere General Medical Center has a bed capacity of 700 as well as 35 bassinets. Last year there were 30,980 adults and children discharged and 2,000 newborn discharges. The hospital has been in existence since 1965 and at the present time, records from 1965 through 1995 have been microfilmed.

The Health Information Management Department is to be relocated next to the Patient Accounts Department in a newly remodeled wing of the hospital. The dimensions of the proposed space allocation are shown on the following diagram (1/16" = 1 foot) as well as the organizational chart for the Health Information Management department. The allocated space is to be prepared according to your specifications.

The following functions are performed by your Health Information Management department:

1. HIM department admission procedure
2. Assembling and discharge analysis of the medical record
3. Statistics (admission, discharge, and required indexes)
4. Release of information and correspondence
5. Dictation and transcription of medical reports (include area for doctors' dictation room)
6. Coding by ICD-9-CM and CPT; abstracting done using an in-house system
7. Numbering and filing (unit number system, terminal digit filing, color-coded folders)
8. Birth certificates
9. Incomplete charts procedure (loose reports, checking charts in physicians' incomplete chart area)
10. Tumor registry
11. DRGs, APCs, and case mix management
12. Utilization management

### Directions:

*For the proposed department, as described, prepare:*

1. A primary layout (1/4" = 1 foot) to consist of the following: Label the physical location of personnel and all equipment based on each function listed above.
2. Overlay drawings and legends consisting of: a) physical aids to communication; i.e., phones, phone jacks, electrical outlets, dictating equipment, etc., and b) lighting scheme.
3. Include in a separate report a typed list of:
   (a) All equipment, furniture, and supplies necessary for each function, and computer hardware and software. Be specific as to type of equipment and dimensions.
   (b) All measurements and calculations used to determine the filing capacity of records in the file area
   (c) Color samples of paint, fabric/carpet, wallpaper, etc. used throughout the department.

*Remember:*   Wall depth = 6"
Door openings = 3'
Decide on dry wall placement (if any) or use of demountable wall panels.

## DIMENSIONS OF PROPOSED LAYOUT
## (SCALE: 1/16" = 1 FOOT)

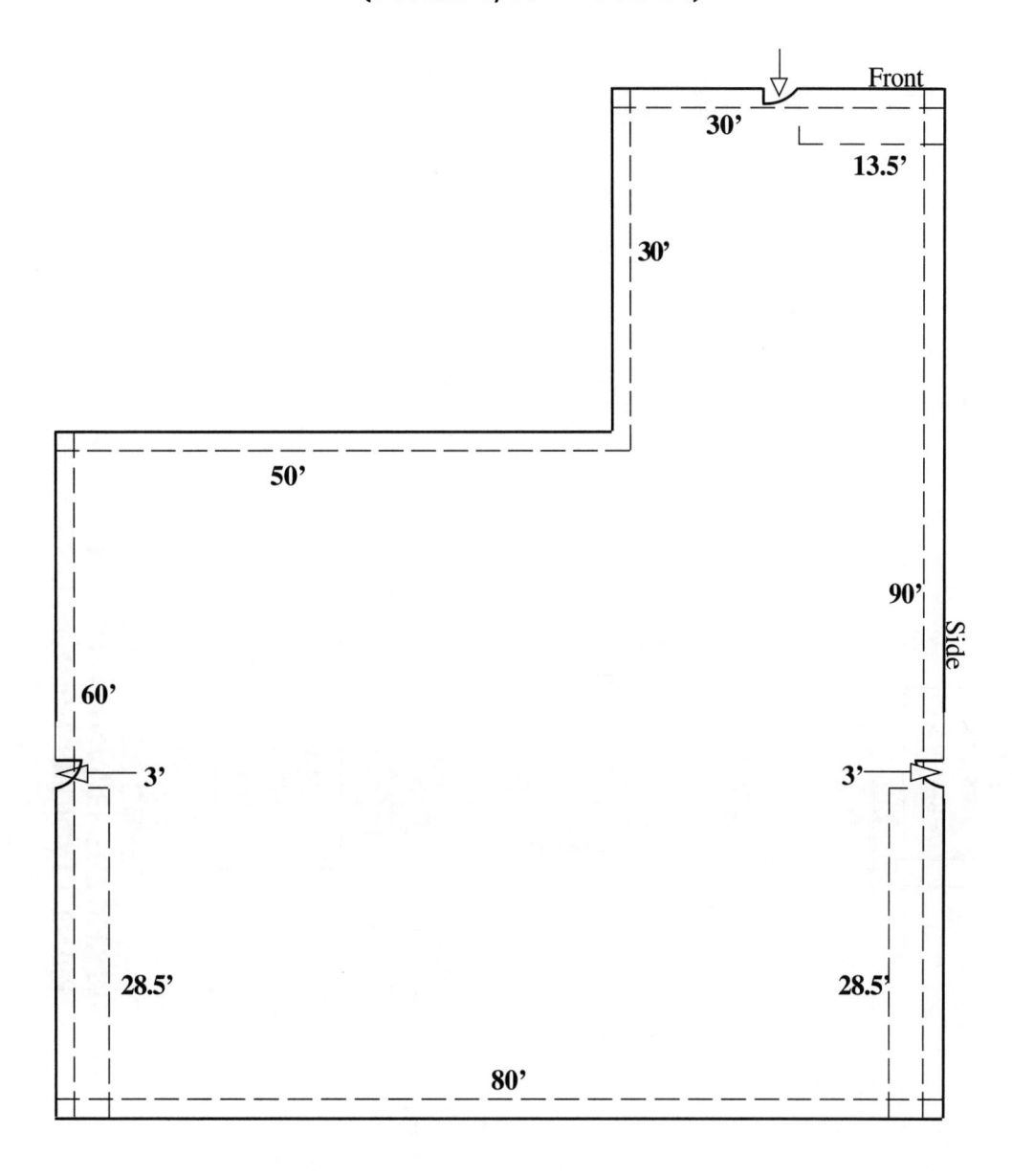

Front

30'

13.5'

30'

50'

90' Side

60'

3'  3'

28.5'  28.5'

80'

Copyright © 2001 by W.B. Saunders Company. All rights reserved.

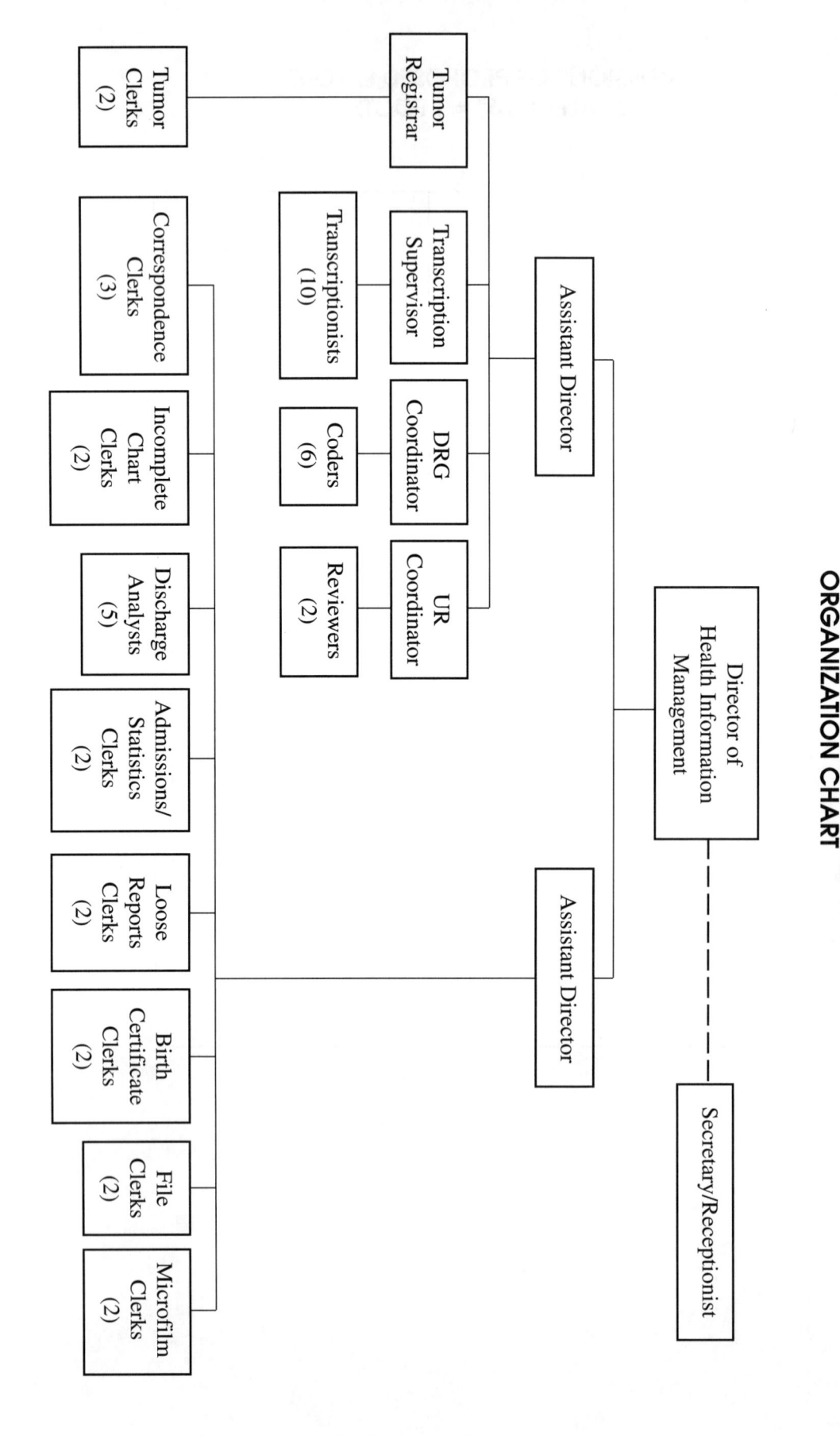

# ANYWHERE GENERAL MEDICAL CENTER
## HEALTH INFORMATION MANAGEMENT DEPARTMENT
### ORGANIZATION CHART

- Director of Health Information Management
  - Secretary/Receptionist (dotted line)
  - Assistant Director
    - Tumor Registrar
      - Tumor Clerks (2)
    - Transcription Supervisor
      - Transcriptionists (10)
    - DRG Coordinator
      - Coders (6)
    - UR Coordinator
      - Reviewers (2)
  - Assistant Director
    - Correspondence Clerks (3)
    - Incomplete Chart Clerks (2)
    - Discharge Analysts (5)
    - Admissions/Statistics Clerks (2)
    - Loose Reports Clerks (2)
    - Birth Certificate Clerks (2)
    - File Clerks (2)
    - Microfilm Clerks (2)

# Review Answers

## PRETEST REVIEW ANSWER KEY

### Directions:

1. Correct your Pretest answers with the answers below by placing a slash through the incorrect question number (Example: 8) with a pen or pencil of a contrasting color.
2. Record the correct answer by placing a square around the letter of the correct answer.
3. Record the total correct on the Initial Performance Grid in Section 4 of this review manual.
4. Calculate your performance rate and also record on the grid.
5. Promptly locate the correct answer for each question missed in the chapter of the textbook.
6. Proceed to the chapter review if your performance rate was 80% or higher; otherwise, return to the chapter for further study.

### Answers to Pretest Review:

| | | | | |
|---|---|---|---|---|
| 1. | d | | 6. | c |
| 2. | a | | 7. | c |
| 3. | b | | 8. | c |
| 4. | d | | 9. | a |
| 5. | b | | 10. | a |

## CHAPTER REVIEW ANSWER KEY

### Directions:

1. Correct your answers with the answers below by placing a slash through the incorrect question number (Example: 8) with a pen or pencil of a contrasting color.
2. Record the correct answer by placing a square around the letter of the correct answer.
3. Record the total correct on the Initial Performance Grid in Section 4 of this review manual.
4. Calculate your performance rate and also record on the grid.
5. Promptly locate the correct answer for each question missed in the chapter of the textbook.
6. Proceed to the next chapter assigned in your study.

### Answers to Chapter Review:

| | | | | |
|---|---|---|---|---|
| 1. | c | | 6. | c |
| 2. | b | | 7. | c |
| 3. | d | | 8. | b |
| 4. | b | | 9. | b |
| 5. | b | | 10. | a |

# CHAPTER 14

# HUMAN RESOURCE MANAGEMENT

## Review

### PRETEST REVIEW

### Directions:

1. Read each question carefully before selecting an answer.
2. Circle the letter of the correct answer.
3. Answer all the questions since there is no penalty for this pretest review.
4. Check your answers with the answer key located at the end of this chapter.

1. The Fair Labor Standards Act makes it illegal to fire an employee for filing a grievance.
   a. True
   b. False

2. Action that follows an infraction is preventive discipline.
   a. True
   b. False

3. The critical incident performance evaluation requires the documentation of good and bad examples of behavior.
   a. True
   b. False

4. The refusal to bargain in good faith with employee representatives constitutes unfair labor activity prohibited by the National Labor Relations Act.
   a. True
   b. False

5. The process of assuring a ready supply of trained help to cover positions when needed is accomplished through job rotation.
   a. True
   b. False

6. A job analysis is a commonly used tool for the development of a Human Resource Plan.
   a. True
   b. False

7. Involuntary termination is the final step in a progressive discipline plan.
   a. True
   b. False

8. A blend of directive and non-directive counseling is called participative employee counseling.
   a. True
   b. False

9. Termination for cause is not grievable.
   a. True
   b. False

10. The elimination of sex-based discrimination in pay practices was mandated by the Fair Labor Standards Act in 1938.
    a. True
    b. False

# CHAPTER REVIEW

## Directions:

1. *Read each question carefully before selecting an answer.*
2. *Circle the letter of the correct answer.*
3. *Answer all the questions since there is no penalty for this pretest review.*
4. *Check your answers with the answer key located at the end of this chapter.*

1. A Human Resource Plan prepares the organization for layoffs.
   a. True
   b. False

2. The halo effect is a performance evaluation rater bias.
   a. True
   b. False

3. Compensation management is regulated by the
   a. JCAHO
   b. National Labor Relations Act
   c. Fair Labor Standards Act
   d. Labor Management Relations Act

4. Attracting qualified applicants is an objective of compensation management.
   a. True
   b. False

5. Employees of state and private hospitals are protected by the Age Discrimination in Employment Act.
   a. True
   b. False

6. The process of fulfilling an organization's mission and goals through human resource management is a functional objective.
   a. True
   b. False

7. New hire screening interviews are generally conducted by the
   a. hiring supervisor
   b. Human Resource Management Department
   c. management
   d. all of the above

8. Affirmative action programs were promulgated by the ADA.
   a. True
   b. False

9. Attrition refers to voluntary resignation or retirement.
   a. True
   b. False

10. Referring to the box on the following page, what is the name of this form?

*Additional review questions can be found on the CD-ROM.*

**Position Title:** Health Information Secretary

**Department:** Health Information Services

**Supervisor:** Manager, Health Information Services

**General Job Objectives:**

1. Acts as department receptionist and first telephone contact.
2. Processes daily work schedules.
3. Coordinates completion and filing of Birth Certificates with Bureau of Vital Statistics.
4. Demonstrates effective relationships with coworkers, patients, public, physicians, administration, and outside agencies.

**Essential Job Duties:**

(List all tasks required to perform the routine functions required for the position.)

Example: Completes birth certificates or fetal death certificates as required. Greets visitors to the department.

Routes incoming phone calls and takes messages when intended party is unavailable.

**Meets Standards of Performance By:** (Example)

(For Greeting Visitors) Receiving no complaints in the performance period concerning discourteous service.

**Exceeds Standards of Performance By:** (Example)

(For Greeting Visitors) Receiving compliments from visitors, coworkers, and physicians on helpfulness and courteous service.

# Assignments

## 14-1: INTEGRATING TELEMEDICAL RECORDS

### Case Study:

Flo Tech, the health information manager, at Upstate University Medical Center, faces a critical challenge in moving her department into the 21st century of health care services. A new telemedicine program has been developed so that rural hospitals can use university specialists as consultants without the patient being transferred. The system transmits digital signals over a wide-band, fiber-optic network, permitting synchronized data and image interactivity. The "record" that results from this interchange includes both a videotape of the interaction between the medical consultant and the on-site health care provider and relevant clinical information extracted from the patient's electronic medical record. The chief executive officer has asked the health information manager to determine how many additional full-time equivalent (FTE) staff, if any, are needed to manage these records.

### Questions:

1. Identify the type of information needed to determine how this new technology will affect current staffing patterns in the department.
2. To use in recruiting and retraining, list the skills, knowledge, and other job specifications needed in the staff that will maintain these types of records.
3. If financial or other constraints preclude adding new staff at this time, what steps should be taken to handle the additional workload?

## 14-2: REDUCTION IN FORCE

### Case Study:

The manager of the HIM department at a 50-bed rural hospital, Page Webb, has a variety of duties, including supervision of the health information management staff. Because of Medicare and Medicaid budget cuts, the hospital lost more than $1 million last year. The hospital administrator announced at a department head meeting that each department must reduce its wage and salary budget by 25 per cent. The HIM department currently employs four full-time individuals, two of whom are single parents with no other source of income. One employee, the spouse of a successful lawyer, works (as she has stated to her supervisor) "just to stay busy." Another employee, a recent graduate of a Health Information Technology (HIT) program, has recently introduced some innovative and cost-saving process changes within the department.

### Questions:

1. What options are available to Ms. Webb to achieve the mandated decrease in wage and salary expenditures?
2. Develop criteria to use in evaluating each of the options that will reduce staff.
3. How should Ms. Webb deal with adverse reactions of the staff anticipated by the necessary RIF (reduction in force)?

## 14-3: ACCOMMODATING GENDER PREFERENCES: SPORTS OR SOAPS?

### Case Study:

Health information services had been an exclusively female domain for as long as the current department director can remember. Last summer, two young male college students were hired for health record analyst positions on the evening shift. Because they exceeded the minimal job qualifications and were available to work immediately, they were hired over several less qualified female applicants. At the most recent HIS supervisors' meeting, the evening supervisor, Stella Latte, expressed a concern about these young men's behavior. Being avid sports fans, they brought a small TV to the office to watch sporting events as they work. Several of the older female employees have complained that the TV was a distraction and stated, "We 'girls' were never allowed to watch our shows on the job." Although organization policy doesn't address this practice, it has been customary for the female employees to operate small radios or CD players discretely on the evening shift, using earphones.

### Questions:

1. Is this issue primarily a gender-based problem? Why or why not?
2. What other factors should be considered in addressing this problem so as to provide a fair and reasonable resolution?
3. How can the concerns of the longer-term employees be addressed to minimize conflict and work disruption?

## 14-4: ENTREPRENEURS WITH MEDICAL LANGUAGE SPECIALISTS

### Case Study:

Health-Are-Us Hospital has made a proposal to offer transcription services of the medical language specialists to a large physician group practice that adjoins the medical center. Dick Tate, the Health Information Management Services manager developed a human resources plan to determine the number of specialists needed and a time line for recruiting, hiring, and training them as a group. He believes that this group processing will be more cost-effective than completing a separate cycle for each new hire, individually. The plan also establishes the process for screening, selecting, and training other hospital employees (non-HIM) as backup staff for HIM functions. Because the volume of medical dictation is likely to flow irregularly, contingency plans for outsourcing transcription are also included. Having developed this staffing plan, Dick Tate feels confident that he can guarantee reliable and uninterrupted services for these physicians.

### Questions:

1. What are the strengths and weaknesses of this staffing approach?
2. Do you share Mr. Tate's confidence in the likely success of this plan? (Explain your response.)
3. What other factors relevant to human resource management should be considered in the development of this staffing plan?

## 14-5: AFFIRMATIVE ACTION IN REVERSE

### Case Study:

A large urban hospital has been required to maintain an affirmative action program because it is a major government contractor ($20 million a year was received from government research contracts and Medicare payments). Under this program, the hospital agreed to promote two women into supervisory positions for each male selected. This promotion practice was to continue until 45 per cent of all the supervisors were women.

Health Information Services had the first open position that qualified under this program, a position as clinical data supervisor. The HIS Director, Dot Calm, was one of the few female department heads in the hospital. This department employs 3 men out of 75 employees. The Director typically asks her Assistant Director, Jack Frost, to participate in the selection process. Frost maintains that a black female employee, Kay G. Ray, is the most qualified for the position. Ray has completed two years in medical school, is a graduate of a bachelor's degree program in health information management, and holds Registered Health Information Administrator (RHIA) and Certified Coding Specialist (CCS) credentials. Also she has worked as a health data analyst in this department for about one year.

Another current employee, Warren Buffer, has also applied for the position. Buffer has nine more years of experience and five more years of seniority in the department than Ms. Ray but does not have comparable educational background or credentials. The human resource specialist recommends that Warren be given the job in compliance with the affirmative action program.

### Questions:

1. What factors should Dot consider in making her final decision?
2. What justification, if any, might she have for not making the affirmative action selection?
3. Which employee would you promote and why?

## 14-6: WORKING WITH UNION EMPLOYEES

### Case Study:

The nonsupervisory employees of the HIM department of Heavenly Days Hospital are included in the bargaining unit representing technical/clerical employees. Donnie Brook, a union member, wants to leave work early to attend her son's Little League baseball game. Donnie informs her supervisor that she agrees to work through her lunch hour so that she will have completed a full eight hours of work that day.

### Questions:

1. What additional information should the supervisor consider before she makes a decision to approve or deny Donnie's request?
2. What problems, if any, might result from her approving this request?
3. What potential benefits might be gained by approving the request?

## 14-7: CHANGES AT HAPPY TRAILS HEALTH CENTER

### Case Study:

Ms. Sippy Delta has just been promoted to manager of health information services at Happy Trails Health Center. A team of physicians, administrators, and department heads has decided to transform the culture of the organization into a quality-driven, patient-centered environment. Health information is stored digitally on optical disk by scanning paper documents. The patient-centered care project calls for a completely electronic health record, with data coming from various sources throughout the organization. Health information services will manage the central data repository. Delta is committed to this innovative approach but is concerned about how to communicate the changes to staff and how the new system will affect the department's operations.

### Questions:

1. What factors should Delta address in implementing this major organizational change?
2. What obstacles is Ms. Delta likely to face as a Department Manager in taking on this project?
3. How can adopting a systems view of human resource management assist the managers responsible for implementing this major change?

## 14-8: IN CASE OF ACCIDENT...

### Case Study:

Generating the physician profiles for reappointment to the medical staff is a demanding responsibility of the HIM Department at Happier Days Memorial Hospital. It involves retrieving and integrating activity statistics and performance data for 450 physicians each year. Virginia Dare, the health data specialist, has coordinated this project for the past several years and has developed an efficient and reliable system for generating accurate and timely reports. The hospital will be adding approximately 35 per cent more physicians next year resulting from its contractual agreements with several large group practices.

Maria Gonzales, the Administrator of Medical Staff Affairs, is responsible for all medical staff credentialing functions. Late one afternoon, she is notified that Virginia has just been seriously injured in an auto accident. Maria's assistant tells her that Virginia is the only one who knows how to complete the profiles. Although written procedures have been established, they are too general and ambiguous for inexperienced staff to follow. The reports must be completed next week to distribute to the clinical staff departments in order to complete the physician credentialing function to facilitate the affiliation process. Ms. Dare's supervisor is quite concerned about this situation since she does not want to give the impression that her HIM Department isn't capable of providing effective and reliable service to her internal clients.

### Questions:

1. Given these circumstances, who (which manager) is responsible for ensuring that this process goes forward with minimal disruption?
2. What should the responsible manager(s) do at this point to minimize the potentially adverse effects of delayed reporting on the operations of the organization and the affiliation of the new physicians?
3. What actions should be taken to anticipate and prevent such a crisis from occurring in the future?

## 14-9: OUT WITH THE OLD AND IN WITH THE NEW

### Case Study:

An integrated management information system was implemented in the Celestial Village Continuum of Care, a 180-bed long-term care facility, owned and operated by a religious order. When Eudora Darling was recruited as Manager of Administrative Systems, she discovered that the technology used in the administrative office was several generations obsolete and that none of the work processes or job functions had been restructured to take full advantage of information technology. Statistics were still being collected manually, and calculations performed by hand-held calculators and adding machines using information from manual entries in daily employee logs. Computer software utilities were available for data base management, electronic spreadsheet and statistical functions, and publication quality reporting. However, the jobs and work processes in the department had to be analyzed and restructured before the staff could take full advantage of this technology (that has become standard in other administrative environments).

### Questions:

1. What issues must Ms. Darling address in achieving effective implementation of the new technology?
2. What outcomes could she reasonably expect to achieve through an effective job analysis process?
3. Should external consultants or internal staff implement this change? Explain your response.

## 14-10: JOB ENRICHMENT OR HARASSMENT?

### Case Study:

An analysis of the coding and insurance positions of the neighborhood health clinic reveals that the insurance clerk could assume some responsibility for coding with the addition of the requirement for basic knowledge of ICD-9-CM and CPT in the job specifications. The clinic often faces a backlog in coding of outpatient service records. Given this job expansion and appropriate training of the staff, the clinic director gains some desirable staffing flexibility while the insurance clerk can obtain additional skills and experience. Not only would this job redesign enhance the facility's capacity to provide more efficient service, but it also might enhance the job satisfaction and career opportunities of employees in this position.

However, the current employee in the insurance clerk position, Gerta Grip, reacted negatively to the proposed job redesign. She claimed that she was being singled out "to be used as a guinea pig" and was being treated unfairly since other employees in the unit had not been asked to take on extra work. Her greatest objection was that her supervisor was trying to expand her workload without a corresponding pay increase. Furthermore, Ms. Grip expressed some anxiety that this new (and unwelcome) attention to her job would result in unfounded allegations that she prolonged her work breaks and took unauthorized smoking breaks.

### Questions:

1. How should Gerta's supervisor respond to her complaints, assuming that she was committed to the job redesign?
2. Do Gerta's concerns have merit? Why or why not?
3. How should her supervisor address any performance-related problems discovered as a consequence of the job analysis?

## 14-11: PHYSICALLY FIT AT ST. EUPHORIA

### Case Study:

Jimmy Bob Beauregard, the Clinical Data Supervisor at St. Euphoria's, an urban community mental health center, noticed in reviewing the clinical coder's job description that it included a physical requirement of being able to lift and carry up to 75 pounds of dead weight. Apparently this related to the occasional need to move boxes of paper records and files from the active file area into an inactive file storage room and place these boxes on the shelves, sometimes above head level. There is no documentation that any applicant had ever been asked to demonstrate this capability during the selection process nor that any employee in this role was ever actually required to do such heavy lifting on the job.

Nonetheless, Jimmy Bob didn't see any harm in retaining this specification in the event it might become useful. Furthermore it could be a useful test of the applicant's general level of fitness, an area about which he had strong feelings. In fact, he decided to request that human resources include this test in their screening process for all nonsupervisory positions in his department.

### Questions:

1. Would you defend Jimmy Bob's decision in this case to retain this job specification? To extend it to other positions in his unit? Explain your response.
2. What legal-regulatory issues should be considered in this case?
3. If management is convinced of the desirability for a fitness requirement for positions in this unit, what must it do to avoid legal challenges?

## 14-12: RECRUITING WITH AN EXECUTIVE SEARCH FIRM

### Case Study:

Martyrs of Managed Care Hospital relies on an executive search firm for providing well-qualified applicants for key managerial and professional positions, especially those for which a nationwide search seems appropriate. The Vice President for Administrative Support Services, Jacque Johnson has placed a top priority upon filling the Director of Health Information Services position without unnecessary delay. The hospital is planning a major information system upgrade and conversion within the next 9 months prior to JCAHO accreditation survey. The search firm's recruiter assigned to this project had not provided Ms. Johnson with any applicants by the end of the first month of the search. Upon her inquiry, the recruiter informed Jacque that the job market was tight for persons with the required skills but that good candidates would be forthcoming soon.

Three weeks later the recruiter sent an e-mail roster of two "well-qualified" candidates followed by their faxed resumes. Ms. Johnson's review of these materials allowed her to conclude quickly that one candidate was at best marginally qualified for this position. The other seemed by experience and current position title to be very well qualified for executive-level financial management positions. Thus it was not clear why this individual had been referred for the position of Director of Health Information Management Services.

### Questions:

1. What factors might have contributed to this recruitment problem?
2. Other than simply terminating the contract and selecting another search firm to restart the process (an option that would likely entail at least another three-four weeks delay), what might Ms. Johnson do to expedite the recruitment process?

## 14-13: EXPLORING NEW SOURCES OF STAFFING

### Case Study:

Rejuvenation Rehabilitation Institute historically has experienced difficulty in attracting competent and dependable entry-level clerical staff for evening, midnight, and Saturday shifts in the Health Information Services Department. The Assistant Director, Rhonda Welsh, who is responsible for hiring and supervising these positions has been asked by a local agency whether there were any positions available for participants in a transitional "Welfare to Work" program. The potential applicants, primarily African-American young to middle-aged mothers with minimal work experience and a high school education, would have completed a six-week "Ready for Work" program at the agency prior to being referred. The agency wanted to identify receptive employers who would participate in a pilot program through a "letter of understanding," which did not require the employer to hire any applicants but would agree to make a good faith effort to consider any applicants referred. If both parties were satisfied six months after initial placements, the agency would offer to negotiate a more formal contract with the employer.

### Questions:

1. What are the potential benefits and costs of this plan from the perspective of the Institute's management?
2. Assuming that Rhonda was enthusiastic about participating in this program, what concerns would she need to address to maximize the likelihood of effective matches with applicants from the agency?
3. What criteria should department management apply in determining the success or failure of this recruitment effort?

## 14-14: WORK SCHEDULE—SET IN STONE?

### Case Study:

Jeri Mander, a tumor registrar, made an appointment to discuss her work schedule with Rose Etta Stone, the Tumor Registry Director. Ms. Mander is nervous about requesting to change her work schedule because Mrs. Stone has a reputation as a "hardliner." Jeri has had the same Sunday through Thursday, daytime schedule for the last five years. In fact this schedule was one of the attractions of this job because it allowed her time to more easily participate in her children's school activities. However, her children are now high school age and she has recently joined a new community church that expects regular participation at worship services and Sunday school. She enjoys her job, has an excellent work record, and doesn't want to jeopardize her position. Yet she feels in a bind because of the priority she gives to her religious obligations.

Consequently she asks her boss to change her schedule to work from Tuesday through Saturday on daytime shift. Ms. Stone is reluctant to make this change since she knows that it is difficult to find staff willing to work on Sundays. However, she also is aware that Jeri is a valuable employee and suspects that some religious freedom issues may be involved. In the interim (while she checks with the HRM Director on any potential legal risks of denying the request), she asks Jeri to present a written request with a justification for the schedule change, an analysis of the impact of the new schedule, and recommendations for dealing with any potential problems associated with it.

### Questions:

1. Assuming that Jeri demonstrates that the schedule change can be accommodated with minimal impact on the work process and output, should Mrs. Stone approve the request? Explain your answer.
2. Under what circumstances relevant to the case might you deny the request?
3. What problems might result by setting this precedent for position-specific scheduling?

# 14-15: DIVERSITY IN THE WORKPLACE

## Case Study:

Abu Okari Al-Amin, an African-American male in his mid-20s, was recently hired by the Health Information Department to manage its photocopying, mailing, and office supplies center. In this role Mr. Al-Amin has regular contact with virtually all of the 25 staff in the department as well as employees and some physicians from other adjacent departments. Mr. Al-Amin is quite articulate, personable, and knowledgeable in his areas of responsibility. However, his long dreadlocks, Afro-Caribbean clothing style, his playing Reggae music on his lunch breaks, and (in the words of one Caucasian employee with 25 years of seniority) his using "militant language" seemed to discomfort or threaten some of the staff.

However, no real problems surfaced until one of the coders, Ms. Joyce Kim, an older Korean-American woman, filed a complaint with her supervisor, Leah Solomon, against Mr. Al-Amin for using "dirty" language in her presence, including the use of ethnic slurs, and otherwise treating her with disrespect. Ms. Kim also claimed that she smelled what she thought might be marijuana when he was close to her. The alleged incidents took place with no other witnesses to corroborate the facts.

Ms. Solomon presented the complaint to Mr. Al-Amin in a one-on-one meeting to give him the opportunity to respond to the charges. Although Mr. Al-Almin conceded that he was not comfortable with Koreans due to tension with Korean businesses in his neighborhood, he denied that he said anything disrespectful or abusive to Ms. Kim. He admitted to using some colorful street language with her that he used regularly with everybody and that no offense had been intended. He brushed off the reference to any drug use.

## Questions:

1. As the employee's supervisor, what steps would you take next to resolve this issue?
2. Assuming that no proven violations of organizational policy were entailed in Mr. Al-Amin's behavior, what further actions, if any, should Ms. Solomon take?
3. What should be done if there are subsequent complaints about Mr. Al-Amin's behavior from other staff?

## 14-16: PERFORMANCE APPRAISAL

### Case Study:

Donna Karan is the director of Health Information Services at Up-Scale Heights Community Medical Center. The medical center has established an objective Performance Appraisal (PA) system based on supervisory ratings in each of five performance dimensions: cooperation, dependability, attitude, quality of work, and quantity of work. The ratings are based on a five point-scale of 1 (unacceptable) to 5 (outstanding). Supervisors are required to provide extensive narrative documentation to justify any ratings of "outstanding." Employees receiving below an overall rating of 3 (average) will not be eligible for consideration for the annual salary increment.

Donna's managers have expressed dissatisfaction with this system because of numerous complaints by employees about perceived unfairness in its administration. In job satisfaction surveys, employees have criticized the PA system as being too subjective and unfair and not very relevant to their jobs. In addition, departmental managers are concerned that this system does not allow for encouragement of continuous improvement in performance.

### Questions:

1. What are the deficiencies in the performance appraisal system as described?
2. What changes would address the concerns raised by management and the employees?
3. How should the revised PA system be implemented to ensure effectiveness?

## 14-17: GUILTY UNTIL PROVEN INNOCENT?

### Case Study:

Molly Maguire, the Director of the HIM Department, came to work early on Saturday morning to find a weekend transcriptionist, Ima Noah Count, slumped over her keyboard apparently asleep or dazed. Molly noticed a thermos at her side that appeared to contain a clear liquid, and smelled a strong odor of alcohol on the employee. Molly aroused Ima from her sleep and told her to leave work immediately and not to return until "you get straight." Although the employee expressed irritation at being interrupted from "her little rest break" and complained about being harassed, she did agree to leave after Molly repeated her order.

Once Ima left the office, Molly, her supervisor, logged on to Ms. Count's e-mail files. Although most of the recent saved entries were routine and work-related, several were messages in an ongoing conversation with an Evelyn who did not have a hospital e-mail address. These messages from Ima were filled with profanity, much of which was directed at Molly, other managers, and fellow employees. In fact, in one message she said "I'd like to get my hands on that fat, nasty @#!!?$@## Molly if she keeps getting on my case again!"

### Questions:

1. How effectively did Molly handle this situation and what might have been done differently in reacting to Ima's behavior under these circumstances?
2. What are the next steps in taking disciplinary action against this employee?
3. Develop a brief policy statement governing e-mail communication that would be relevant to the issues in this case.

## 14-18: OVERZEALOUS AND UNDERDRESSED

### Case Study:

Tanya Tuckerman, an information system analyst, works closely with the physicians in data management and distribution on the 3:00 to 11:00 PM shift. She has an excellent work record and meets all the productivity standards specified in her job description. Barbara Bushwhack, the day shift supervisor who works 8:30 AM to 5:00 PM, became Tanya's supervisor when the night shift supervisor was eliminated in a cost control effort. She monitors Tanya's performance by reviewing her documentation and meeting with her periodically but doesn't interact with Tanya a great deal because of their different schedules.

Barbara has noticed that occasionally Tanya has dressed inappropriately, too provocative for business attire. She realizes that Tanya has not technically violated the departmental dress code, although in her opinion she "pushes the limit." Recently, Barbara was contacted by a female resident physician to complain that Tanya had been "falling all over" several of the male residents and often made inappropriate, suggestive comments to them in response to their "joking around." The female resident felt offended by these displays and was increasingly uncomfortable with what she considered to be Tanya's "flaunting it." The resident was so upset about this situation that she promised to file a grievance with the Medical Director if the situation wasn't corrected without delay.

Barbara assured the resident that she would address the situation right away and report back to her within several days. In considering how to handle this situation, she recognized that this was not the first time that physicians have complained about Tanya's behavior as being "unprofessional." Tanya's personnel file included a note from the former evening supervisor who at least once advised Tanya about adopting "more professional dress and attitudes" while at work.

### Questions:

1. What actions should Ms. Bushwhack take to resolve this situation effectively and fairly?
2. What other information, if any, should Barbara obtain to take more informed action?
3. What supervisory/managerial issues might have contributed to the problems resulting from Tanya's alleged behavior?

## 14-19: WORK FROM HOME: WILL IT WORK?

### Case Study:

Willie "the Web" Wonk was hired as a Web design specialist and Internet trouble-shooter for the Information Services and Telecommunications Division of Merger Mania Medical Center. As a highly skilled, very independent self-starter, Mr. Wonk negotiated a flexible work schedule that allowed him to complete much of his work at his home office so long as he was available "on call" by e-mail or telephone and he maintained on-site hours for two half-days each week. His supervisor, the Assistant Director of the IS&T Division, Electra Nett, was very pleased with Willie's progress on the redesign of the organization's Web presentation and his willingness to take new initiatives.

The scheduling arrangement seemed to be working smoothly for the first three months of his employment, but recently Ms. Nett has had some concerns. Several of the department chairs (as Mr. Wonk's internal clients) had complained about their staff not being able to reach Willie to address immediate problems. Worse yet, he often would not respond to their e-mail or phone messages until the next workday or later. Although none of these problems could reasonably be considered crises, the affected staff was increasingly impatient with these delays and the implicit lack of priority given to their problems suggested by Willie's unresponsiveness. Although Ms. Nett had preferred to meet with him during his on-site hours, Willie had left her a message that he would not be in the office at all this week but could be reached by e-mail. With some irritation, Electra decided to call him directly to arrange a meeting ASAP. After several rings she received a message that "this number had been disconnected and the forwarding number was unlisted at the customer's request."

### Questions:

1. What should Electra do next to address this situation?
2. Do you believe that the original scheduling arrangement was reasonable? Why or why not?
3. Should this situation be treated through the regular performance appraisal system or as a disciplinary matter? Explain your response.

## 14-20: JOB EVALUATION

### Case Study:

The Health Information Services Department has some of the lowest salary ranges in the hospital. Samantha Surfeit, the Department Director, is concerned with the increasing dissatisfaction expressed by the data management staff concerning their pay level. One especially outspoken employee, Ron Righteous, who claimed to speak for the whole unit, argued that employees in these positions must have excellent technical skills and training to perform to expectations. Furthermore, they typically work under stress of heavy workloads and deadlines and are frequently expected to stay beyond their normal quit times to complete urgent work or cover for employees who are on leave. In spite of these demands and high levels of performance, the data management staff on average do not earn as much as medical secretaries in the clinical units of the hospital.

Although Samantha takes these concerns of her staff quite seriously, she realizes that she cannot resolve them independently. Consequently, she contacts the Director of Human Resources, Bonita Benefactor, to enlist her support to address the apparent salary inequities. The HR Director offers to complete a "quick and dirty" salary analysis to compare the pay of these staff with comparable positions elsewhere in the hospital, including the medical secretaries. Several days later she informs Samantha that the medical secretarial positions are earning approximately $1.75 per hour more on average than data management staff positions. Bonita also indicates that she does not have the resources at this time to do a more formal organization-wide compensation analysis, nor can she realistically anticipate that one would be possible in the foreseeable future. Consequently, she advises Samantha to examine the job descriptions of her staff to determine whether they accurately reflect the skills, knowledge, and scope and level of responsibility for these positions. However, the HR Director is not very encouraging about the prospects of any action in the current budget year to address any identified compensation inequities.

### Questions:

1. Under the circumstances, what would be the likely benefits of completing the suggested job evaluation?
2. Assuming that Samantha can demonstrate that the skills, knowledge, and responsibilities of her staff are comparable to or higher than other staff in the hospital that are more highly compensated, what action should be taken to address this problem in the long term?
3. What can Samantha do, if anything, to respond to her employees' concerns and dissatisfaction in the short term?

## 14-21: SYSTEMS MODEL OF HUMAN RESOURCE MANAGEMENT

### Assignment:

1. Using a diagram with labels and arrows, explain the basic relationships among the core functions and activities of human resources management.
2. Identify which of the functions discussed in Chapter 14 in the text is most central to the whole system. Explain your response.

## 14-22: PROFESSIONAL PRACTICE: JOB ANALYSIS

### Assignment:

1. Based on Chapter 14 in the text and any relevant work experience, outline eight (8) key activities of the job analysis process for a health information services environment.
2. Identify a professional practice experience site where the supervisor will allow you to conduct a pilot implementation of your job analysis process for one or more jobs in the unit.
3. Implement this process and document your results, identifying specific job requirements, essential functions (per the Americans With Disabilities Act), and job specifications (for use in employee selection).

## 14-23: JOB DESCRIPTIONS

### Assignment:

1. Critique and revise the job description on the following page to make it a more useful and valid document. Identify and supply any relevant information that is omitted. Reword and clarify any language that is unclear, inconsistent, or inappropriate.
2. Indicate briefly how the revised job description might be effectively used for the following human resource management functions:
   A. Employee selection
   B. Orientation
   C. Performance appraisal
   D. Compensation management.
3. Make a brief but convincing argument for or against the following claim:

   "Given the trends toward increasing organizational flexibility, employee demands for participation, and the need for ongoing learning and adaptation with the dramatic impact of information technology in the workplace, the traditional job description has become obsolete and should be abandoned. Preparing and revising job descriptions is simply a waste of time and effort."

# Health Information Department
# Job Description

Position: Manager
Reports to: Director

## Summary

This person is under the direct supervision of the Director of the Department. He must be familiar with all jobs in his department

## Work and Duties

1. Supervises sections of the Health Records Department under his direction. This individual will act as Acting Director on as needed basis.
2. Directs the operation of Medical Records as delegated by his supervisor by assigning and scheduling the work of the various staff.
3. The Director delegates activities for ongoing and continuing monitoring within the unit.
4. Organizes, plans, and implements a system to insure that all complete files are maintained properly and that missing files are located.
5. Meetings with administrative supervisors as needed.
6. Responsible for various responsibilities for Medical Records orientation and training for new employees and others.
7. Assists with chart completion procedures and coding validation (occasionally).
8. Liaison for the department with attorneys requesting medical record information, subpoenas and court orders, and/or give testimony.
9. Maintains a schedule of performance and potential review dates for Medical Record employees and determines related performance evaluations under the guidance of the Director. Suggests salary increases related to performance evaluations and recommends training, promotion, transfer or disciplinary actions except for terminations. Makes some decisions in Director's absence.
10. Vacation and holiday schedules.
11. Microfilming and storage issues.
12. Oversight of the filing/retention/retrieval of Outpatient Department records.
13. Performs ongoing functions of information dissemination and processing and provides query triage, compilation, adjudication, validation, and documentation relative to professional standards and criteria as well as relevant organization-wide policies and procedures.
14. Reviews and approves time cards.

## Qualifications for the Job

This person must have good organizational skills and a good attitude. He should be able to control his employees in a firm and efficient manner.

## Authorization

I agree that this is a full and complete list of all required duties and activities for this individual.

Supervisor: _____

## 14-24: HUMAN RESOURCES PLANNING AND FORECASTING

### Assignment:

1. Describe and explain the process to follow for estimating both supply of and demand for nonprofessional and technical staff in a health information department.
2. In what ways, if any, might the process differ for managerial and professional positions? Explain your response.
3. Provide a brief explanation of the following concepts and tools relevant to human resource planning and forecasting:
    A. Reconciliation
    B. Staffing table
    C. Replacement chart
    D. Skill inventory
4. What factors in the health care environment are most likely to affect the organization's capacity to conduct effective human resource planning in the new millennium?

## 14-25: EMPLOYEE SELECTION PROCESS

### Assignment:

*Identify strengths and deficiencies of the following process used to select information analysts in a large health information support services department at Metro University Medical Center. Provide specific recommendations for how and why the process should be improved.*

### Selection Process:

Due to the highly competitive market for information analysts with Web design skills, the Medical Center offers a $100 bonus to any employee referring a qualified applicant. Human Resources staff screens applications both paper-based and electronic. Applicants who meet basic eligibility criteria for education and work experience are referred to the Department Head. She reviews them quickly, shares them with the Assistant Director, and then selects the top four candidates to be interviewed. These applicants are contacted to schedule interviews and a mandatory physical exam.

The Director and Assistant Director each interview two of the applicants for the position if her/his schedule permits. Applicants in the final screening group who cannot be conveniently scheduled for interviews are kept in the pool until the final decision is made.

The interview process consists of a loosely structured interview based on the information on the application or resume. The Director requests the Assistant Director's recommendations of his preferred and next best candidates. Pending positive written responses from the selected applicant's references, the Director makes the final decision and notifies the Human Resources staff.

## 14-26: EMPLOYEE ORIENTATION AND RETENTION

### Assignment:

Excessive employee turnover can be a major problem, with its potentially adverse effects on productivity, stability, and employee morale. Often turnover in health care is greatest for those jobs characterized by low pay, routine (nonchallenging) work, and limited prospects for career mobility without increased education and professional credentials, e.g., filing clerks, nursing home aides. Develop a strategy for improving employee retention (or decreasing turnover) by responding to the following questions.

1. How does an effective orientation program enhance employee retention?
2. Develop a plan of activities for a 1-day orientation program for nonprofessional employees in a health information department, assuming two 3-hour sessions. Specify the activities that would occur at the various times of day, e.g., 8 to 10 AM: _____.
3. Outline the key points that need to be included during the initial orientation of new employees. Be sure to address both departmental and organization-wide issues.
4. Describe how the effectiveness of this employee orientation can be measured.

## 14-27: PERFORMANCE APPRAISAL SYSTEM

### Case Study:

The performance appraisal process at a large community hospital consists of:

- Annual completion of an Employee Evaluation Form (see the following) by the immediate supervisor
- A brief (lasting between 5 to 10 minutes) formal appraisal interview, when the supervisor reviews the information on the form with the employee and asks for comments

This process is always scheduled during the last month of the fiscal year so that the salary adjustment decisions are included in the following budget year. In the event of the supervisor or employee's illness or an unavoidable scheduling problem, the supervisor may forward the appraisal form to the Human Resources Department with a copy sent to the employee. Then the formal performance review session is waived.

### Employee Satisfaction Survey Data:

The following data from an employee satisfaction survey completed within the past 2 years addresses performance appraisal:

1. Do you believe that the performance evaluation system is fairly administered?
   **Yes: 10%**    **No: 60%**    **Uncertain: 30%**
2. How helpful is the annual performance review with your supervisor in providing feedback for improvement?
   **Very Helpful: 5%**   **Of Some Help: 15%**   **Of No Help: 60%**
   **No Performance Review Scheduled: 20%**
3. Are you satisfied that your compensation fairly represents your level of performance and contributions?
   **Yes: 15%**    **No: 75%**    **Uncertain: 10%**

## Questions:

1. Identify and discuss specific strengths and deficiencies of the Employee Evaluation Form.
2. Discuss any other deficiencies in the current performance appraisal process (in addition to any associated with the rating form).
3. List the recommendations you would suggest to improve the effectiveness of this performance appraisal process.

# Really Good Health Care Center
# Employee Evaluation Form

**Employee's Name:** _____          **Job Title:** _____

*Mark an X at the point on the scale that corresponds to your best judgment about the employee's effectiveness for each performance component.*

|  | Poor |  | Average |  | Excellent |
|---|---|---|---|---|---|
| Cooperativeness | 1 | 2 | 3 | 4 | 5 |
| Dependability | 1 | 2 | 3 | 4 | 5 |
| Accuracy | 1 | 2 | 3 | 4 | 5 |
| Attitude | 1 | 2 | 3 | 4 | 5 |
| Loyalty | 1 | 2 | 3 | 4 | 5 |
| Quantity of Work | 1 | 2 | 3 | 4 | 5 |
| Quality of Work | 1 | 2 | 3 | 4 | 5 |
| Overall Performance | 1 | 2 | 3 | 4 | 5 |

## Recommendations

I recommend the following salary adjustment for the next budget year:     $ _____

Supervisor: _____          Date: _____

Copyright © 2001 by W.B. Saunders Company. All rights reserved.

## 14-28: COMPENSATION MANAGEMENT FOR TEAMS

### Background:

Developing fair and effective compensation policies and processes for teams is a major challenge. The use of team-based work is growing in virtually all industries. Typically the team structure is flexible and membership is fluid, with its life lasting as long as the project or task, e.g., 3 to 18 months. Team leaders may be chosen in a variety of ways: appointed, chosen by the team itself, and/or rotated among the members. Team roles and responsibilities may be explicitly established at the outset, or these may evolve as the team members define the problem(s) and develop their own structure and division of responsibilities.

Regardless of the degree of structure and formalization of the team organization, results of the team's efforts must be recognized at least in part as resulting from teamwork, the coordinated contributions of a group. This fact complicates the attempt to provide equitable and effective compensation for team members, not to mention others who support the team efforts but are external to it. The key questions to be faced are:

- How are team members fairly rewarded for their differential talents and contributions while recognizing the team as a whole and its investment in the project?
- How is an effective level of employee satisfaction and motivation maintained for future efforts?

*Address these issues by making general recommendations for effective compensation in the following scenario.*

### Scenario: Information System Integration and Development (ISID) Team

The CEO of Restoration Right Rehabilitation (RRR) Center, Ms. Dot Org, has established a multidisciplinary project team to develop a plan for the design and implementation of a comprehensive information system upgrade and integration. It is anticipated that the project will take 12 to 15 months for completion of:

- An electronic rehabilitation clinical record system (currently in development)
- Linkages between the clinical, billing, budgeting, and quality improvement databases
- Web-based decision support utilities

## ISID Project Team

| Name | Job Title | Time/Effort | Salary |
|---|---|---|---|
| Cora D. Nador | IS Design Manager<br>Project Team Leader | 60% | $105,600 |
| Beverly Binary | Data Manager | 75 | 85,250 |
| Al G. Rhythm | Lead Programmer | 75 | 72,125 |
| C.S. "Tim" Query | IS Analyst | 100 | 68,475 |
| Jill Java | Web Designer | 50 | 60,275 |
| Don Dooright | Human Resource Spec. | 25 | 55,725 |
| Sally Scribe | Technical Writer | 30 | 50,675 |
| Ima Drudge | Admin. Secretary | 50 | 32,550 |

## Compensation System:

The RRR Center has had a traditional (individual performance-based) compensation system with an annual cost of living adjustment (COLA) granted for all satisfactory employees and a merit performance pool of 5 per cent of total base salary budget reserved for exceptional performance. These salary adjustments are subject to the Center's achieving its annual profit margin target and other financial objectives. A merit pay committee representing department heads and top management competitively awards recommendations for merit increases made by department heads with justification. The Center has not previously considered recognizing team-based achievement in its compensation plan.

## Assignment:

1. Given the general characteristics and constraints presented above, develop a plan for an equitable and effective compensation for project teams on a pilot basis.
2. Identify the problems and concerns that should be addressed in the design and implementation of the plan. (Assume that a COLA of 2.25 percent and a merit pool of 3.0 percent will be available in the target year for the employees overall.)

## 14-29: PROGRESSIVE EMPLOYEE DISCIPLINE

## Assignment:

1. Support or reject the following claim by a patient billing supervisor:

    "When an employee crosses the line, she should be dealt with soon and strictly. There should be no excuse at all for any uncertainty about the reasons for the punishment and how it will be carried out. Pampering problem employees just leads to worse problems down the line. When an employee breaks the rules, act first and then explain later. No delays and no regrets ... and you'll have fewer headaches!"

2. Explain what is "progressive" about a progressive discipline process.

3. What are the advantages of immediate suspension of an employee in response to an especially serious or chronic breach of conduct or policy? What, if any, might be the disadvantages?

## 14-30: CAREER PLANNING AND DEVELOPMENT

## Assignment:

1. Develop a career plan for yourself that includes the following items:
    A. Goals
       - Short-term (within 1 year)
       - Mid-term (1 year to 5 years)
       - Long-term (beyond 5 years)
    B. Personal strengths (What am I proud of?)
    C. Areas for personal hrowth (How can I be/do better?)
    D. Specific skills, knowledge and abilities (What strengths can I build on?)
    E. Education and training required (What other tools do I need to achieve my goals?)
    F. How will I know if and when I've achieved my ultimate career goal(s)?

2. What are the major responsibilities of the immediate supervisor in the training and development of her employees?

3. Should the supervisor play a role in the long-term career planning of the employee, or is this primarily the employee's concern? If the supervisor should be involved, how can she do so effectively?

4. Consider the following comments of a middle manager concerning his employees' career development:

    "I am committed to ensuring that all my employees work their way out of their jobs, that most are in the process of preparing to leave for greener pastures and greater challenges. This makes for some uncertainty and short-term adjustments, but in the long term I'll have more productive and more satisfied employees overall."

    Explain why you essentially agree or disagree with this position.

Chapter 14: Human Resource Management ■ 255

# Review Answers

## PRETEST REVIEW ANSWER KEY

### Directions:

1. Correct your Pretest answers with the answers below by placing a slash through the incorrect question number (Example: *8*) with a pen or pencil of a contrasting color.
2. Record the correct answer by placing a square around the letter of the correct answer.
3. Record the total correct on the Initial Performance Grid in Section 4 of this review manual.
4. Calculate your performance rate and also record on the grid.
5. Promptly locate the correct answer for each question missed in the chapter of the textbook.
6. Proceed to the chapter review if your performance rate was 80% or higher; otherwise, return to the chapter for further study.

### Answers to Pretest Review:

| | | | | |
|---|---|---|---|---|
| 1. | b | | 6. | b |
| 2. | b | | 7. | a |
| 3. | a | | 8. | a |
| 4. | a | | 9. | a |
| 5. | a | | 10. | b |

## CHAPTER REVIEW ANSWER KEY

### Directions:

1. Correct your answers with the answers below by placing a slash through the incorrect question number (Example: *8*) with a pen or pencil of a contrasting color.
2. Record the correct answer by placing a square around the letter of the correct answer.
3. Record the total correct on the Initial Performance Grid in Section 4 of this review manual.
4. Calculate your performance rate and also record on the grid.
5. Promptly locate the correct answer for each question missed in the chapter of the textbook.
6. Proceed to the next chapter assigned in your study.

### Answers to Chapter Review:

| | | | | |
|---|---|---|---|---|
| 1. | b | | 6. | b |
| 2. | a | | 7. | a |
| 3. | c | | 8. | b |
| 4. | a | | 9. | a |
| 5. | a | | 10. | job analysis |

Copyright © 2001 by W.B. Saunders Company. All rights reserved.

# CHAPTER 15

# FINANCIAL MANAGEMENT

## Review

### PRETEST REVIEW

### Directions:
1. *Read each question carefully before selecting an answer.*
2. *Circle the letter of the correct answer.*
3. *Answer all the questions since there is no penalty for this pretest review.*
4. *Check your answers with the answer key located at the end of this chapter.*

1. An organization's equity and liabilities are located on its balance sheet.
    a. True
    b. False

2. The proposed outlay for an automated Master Patient Index would be found in the capital budget.
    a. True
    b. False

3. The management tool that predicts when cash will be received and dispersed is a chart of accounts.
    a. True
    b. False

4. The specific budget that determines sources and uses of cash is called the operating budget.
    a. True
    b. False

5. The proposed outlay for a DRG Encoder would be found in the operating budget.
    a. True
    b. False

6. Estimating gross operating revenues is a major phase in developing the Business Plan.
    a. True
    b. False

7. On April 1, Rocky Mountain Hospital is obligated to pay the final balance of $2,500 for the purchase of new PCs. The amount owed is considered a liability.
    a. True
    b. False

8. FTE expenses are figured in the operating budget.
    a. True
    b. False

9. The accrual accounting method records revenues as they are received.
   a. True
   b. False

10. The denominator for calculating current ratio is current liabilities.
    a. True
    b. False

# CHAPTER REVIEW

## Directions:

1. Read each question carefully before selecting an answer.
2. Circle the letter of the correct answer.
3. Answer all the questions since there is no penalty for this pretest review.
4. Check your answers with the answer key located at the end of this chapter.

1. The balance displays all of the following *except:*
   a. assets
   b. equity
   c. liabilities
   d. revenues

2. An organization can measure its ability to meet its short- and long-term obligations by calculating its:
   a. capitalization ratio
   b. liquidity ratio
   c. both a and b
   d. neither a nor b

3. When the current ratio is 3:1:
   a. the payback period is 3 years
   b. the: amount of cash and liquid assets needed to meet bills is three times what is needed
   c. the expense required to supply needed revenue will be three times the net revenue
   d. a 3% return on your investment will be realized

4. Which budgeting approach requires a description of consequences if health care programs or services are terminated or reduced?
   a. rolling
   b. zero-based
   c. flexible
   d. both b and c

5. Rocky Mountain Hospital wants to evaluate how well its resources are being used for the new Sports Medicine Clinic. Which ratio analysis would supply the needed information?
   a. activity ratio
   b. current ratio
   c. capitalization ratio
   d. operating margin ratio

6. Rocky Mountain Health Information Services Department purchased five automobiles for use in delivering records from its centralized location to the twenty clinics it serves in the community. Each of the clinics has an option of hiring its own courier to deliver and retrieve mail sent to the central location or use the Health Information Services delivery vehicle. Each clinic has chosen to use the Health Information Services option. Each car cost $12,000 and has an estimated useful life of three years.

    The Accounting Department uses straight line depreciation. The Health Information Services Department anticipates that each car will be used to make 1,500 mail deliveries per year. For each mail delivery there will be a charge of $3.00 that can be applied toward a future purchase of a replacement vehicle. What is the payback period for the cars?

## Rocky Mountain Hospital
## Balance Sheet
## 12/31/9X

| Assets | 199X |
|---|---|
| Current Assets* | $ 2,438,776 |
| Fixed Assets | 5,874,231 |
| Other Assets | 558,432 |
| Total Assets | $ 8,871,439 |

**Liabilities and Fund Balances**

| | |
|---|---|
| Current Liabilities | |
|     Accounts and notes payable | $345,798 |
|     Staffing and payroll-related | 841,621 |
|     Other short-term payables | 10,102 |
| Total Current Liabilities | $ 1,197,521 |
| Long-Term Liabilities | |
|     Long-term debt | $5,950,728 |
|     Note payable | 2,000,000 |
| Total Long-Term Liabilities | $ 7,950,728 |
| Total Liabilities | $9,148,249 |
| Fund Balance | $ (276.810) |
| Total Liabilities and Fund Balance | $ 8,871,439 |

*Includes $1,438,776 in patient accounts receivable

## Rocky Mountain Hospital
## Income Statement
## 1/1/9X-12/31/9X

| Revenues from Operations | 199X |
|---|---|
| Patient Services | $2,855,500 |
| Less Contractual Allowances | 24,645 |
| Net Patient Service: Revenue | $2,830,865 |
| Net Other Revenues | 123,744 |
| Total Revenue from Operations | $2,954,609 |

**Expenses form Operations**

| | |
|---|---|
| Salaries and Expenses | $1,124,818 |
| Management Salaries and Expenses | 305,720 |
| Other Salaries and Expenses | 213,412 |
| Supplies and Books | 486,257 |
| Utilities | 38,110 |
| Depreciation | 542,333 |
| Interest and Other | 305 124 |
| Total Expenses from Operations | $3,015,774 |

7. Referring to the information in the tables on the previous page, compute the current ratio.

8. Referring to the information in the tables on the previous page, compute the operating margin ratio.

9. A free-standing ambulatory care center incurs medical record folder costs of $3 per new patient and has a monthly rent payment on its space of $12,000. Which of these is a variable cost?

10. Referring to the information in question #9, which is a fixed cost?

*Additional review questions can be found on the CD-ROM.*

# Assignments

## 15-1: COSTS PLANNING

### Scenario:

A family practice physician who has just completed her residence is considering the cost of doing business as a solo practitioner. She needs to determine the costs of doing business.

### Questions:

1. List the types of expenses associated with the solo physician's office, i.e., rental of space.
2. Categorize each type of expense in Question 1 as fixed, variable, or semivariable.
3. Estimate the likely costs of doing business in your city as a family practitioner in a solo practice on an annual basis.
4. Estimate the annual patient service revenue needed to stay in business.
5. Relate revenue to the amount of service possible by one physician.
6. Describe how the financial picture changes in fee for service vs. capitation environments.
7. Where might cost benefits occur if the family physician teamed up with two or three other physicians? What are the negative consequences of this idea?

## 15-2: GRAPHIC REPRESENTATION OF DATA AND DATA ANALYSIS

Using the following data (or data supplied by your instructor) create one or more graphic presentations to present these data to the Hospital Surgery Committee.

1. Calculate the Cost per Case and the Cost per Minute for each month.
2. List the questions the data analysis raises. What other data resources are available in a hospital to answer these questions?
3. Before developing the graphics, determine the key points to reference in the graphics and to use during the presentation.

### Anesthesia Supply Cost per Minute Analysis

| Month | Total Cost | Surgical Cases | Cost per Case | Total Minutes | Cost per Minute |
|---|---|---|---|---|---|
| June | 9,883 | 255 | | 10,000 | |
| July | 11,555 | 245 | | 12,500 | |
| August | 13,350 | 235 | | 13,500 | |
| September | 14,750 | 225 | | 15,300 | |
| October | 16,330 | 215 | | 16,700 | |
| November | 17,400 | 205 | | 17,800 | |

Copyright © 2001 by W.B. Saunders Company. All rights reserved.

## 15-3: DETERMINING THE COST OF PROCESSING REQUESTS FOR INFORMATION

Determine the cost of processing requests for information using the following data.

| Type of Requests | Average Time to Respond to Request |
| --- | --- |
| In-person requests: Someone appears in the Patient Data Services/HIM Department and requests to review and/or receive copies of the record | 15 minutes |
| Requests received by mail or by fax | 8 minutes |
| Requests received by telephone | 5 minutes |

*One FTE (2080 hours) is assigned to this function.*
*The salary for this position is $29,000 a year.*

### Questions:

1. What is the unit cost of the time to respond to requests for information?
2. What other data should be factored into this cost to obtain a unit cost for this function?
3. Given the following mix of types of requests, approximately how many requests could be answered per year? (e.g., 50% mail/fax, 25% telephone, and 25% in person)

## 15-4: STAFFING BUDGET USING PRODUCTIVITY INFORMATION

Helper Hospital has 350 beds with active ED and 20,000 outpatient clinic visits a year.

### Helper Hospital
### Health Information Management Services
### Productivity Data

| Task | Average Time in Minutes |
|---|---|
| Release of information | 25 |
| Pull record | 2 |
| Transport record to ED | 3 |
| Assemble—inpatient record | 5 |
| Assemble—outpatient record | 1.5 |
| File inpatient loose sheet | 0.8 |
| File outpatient loose sheet | 0.6 |
| Code inpatient record<br>  LOS 1–4 days<br>  LOS 5–8<br>  LOS 9–12<br>  LOS 13–25 | <br>13<br>20<br>28<br>42 |
| Code outpatient/ED record | 4 |

### Questions:

1. What other functions need time values assigned?
2. How much detail should be included in the task list?
3. What other methods might be used to estimate/justify FTE?
4. What data from the previous year/months are likely available to help associate HIM productivity data with overall business data/activity data at this facility?

## 15-5: VARIANCE ANALYSIS

1. Use the following information about supply consumption to determine the usage and price variances. The department is considered to be 100 percent variable with volume. Actual units of service were 8,100 compared with a budget of 9,000.

| Supplies | Usage Actual | Usage Budget | Dollar Amounts Actual | Dollar Amounts Budget |
|---|---|---|---|---|
| Item A | 1,780 | 750 | 7,920 | 2,625 |
| Item B | 1,600 | 1,599 | 8,578 | 6,972 |
| Item C | 1,500 | 1,524 | 4,500 | 4,983 |
| Item D | 400 | 411 | 740 | 748 |
| Item E | 450 | 426 | 89,100 | 83,164 |
| Item F | 100 | 180 | 1,600 | 2,740 |
| Item G | 74 | 93 | 2,109 | 2,655 |
| Item H | 350 | 348 | 8,747 | 8,707 |
| Item I | 30 | 30 | 2,250 | 2,245 |
| Item J | 120 | 114 | 8,120 | 5,792 |
| Total | | | 131,692 | 120,631 |

2. Use variance analysis to determine the cause(s) of the salary variance. The department is considered 60 percent variable.

|  | Actual | Budget |
|---|---|---|
| Salaries | 457,600 | 474,240 |
| Paid Hours | 41,600 | 39,520 |
| Volume | 66,500 | 70,000 |

3. A new procedure can be offered at a price of $1,400. The patient population is anticipated to be 80 percent commercially insured patients and 20 percent self-pay. The expected collection rates are 90 percent for commercial insurance and 100 percent for self-pay. Each procedure consumes $288 of supplies. Fixed costs are anticipated to be $765,000. What is the break-even point?

## 15-6: CASE MIX ANALYSIS

### Scenario:

The hospital's Chief Executive Officer anticipates preliminary discussions with three different managed care organizations for the purpose of contracting the facility's surgery product line. In preparation for these initial discussions and to negotiate successful agreements, the CEO needs the information listed below. (Confine analysis to the inpatient population by DRG.)

### Directions:

Using the data in the following tables:

1. Determine a case mix index by payer.
2. Display variance information by length of stay (LOS) and by reimbursement/charges.
3. Determine if the following is a financially sound move: If the facility reduces the price by 20 percent and reduces fixed costs by 10 percent while Olympic guarantees 100 more cases in this product line (assume 15 percent mark-up.)
4. Prepare a report including tables from Questions 1 and 2 above and recommendations for the focus of strategic planning and marketing efforts. Include in the report other data/information/considerations that might need to be factored into the recommendations. List all assumptions used in the analysis and/or recommendations.

### DRG Information

| DRG # | Description | Weight | National LOS |
|---|---|---|---|
| 195 | Cholecystectomy w/CDE w/CC | 2.1972 | 5.6 |
| 196 | Cholecystectomy w/CDE w/o CC | 1.5861 | 4.9 |
| 197 | Cholecystectomy w/o CDE w/CC | 1.5280 | 4.6 |
| 198 | Cholecystectomy w/o CDE w/o CC | 1.0086 | 3.8 |

*(Consult Federal Register/Grouper manuals for actual weight and LOS values.)*

## Hospital Reimbursement Conversion Factors

| Payer | Conversion Factor |
|---|---|
| Cascade | $1000 |
| Olympic | $1050 |
| Columbia | $950 |

## Hospital Costs

**Surgery Product Line: Olympic**

| | | |
|---|---|---|
| cost per case | $1200 | |
| price per case | $1380 | (15% mark-up) |
| fixed cost | $180,000 | |
| variable cost | $480 | per case |

## Payer Information

| DRG | Payer | Number of Patients | Average LOS | Average Charges |
|---|---|---|---|---|
| 195 | Cascade | 130 | 5.6 | $2430 |
| 196 | Cascade | 125 | 4.9 | $1765 |
| 197 | Cascade | 35 | 4.6 | $1495 |
| 198 | Cascade | 260 | 3.8 | $945 |
| 195 | Olympic | 40 | 6.0 | $2420 |
| 196 | Olympic | 120 | 5.1 | $1750 |
| 197 | Olympic | 15 | 5.1 | $1510 |
| 198 | Olympic | 75 | 4.5 | $940 |
| 195 | Columbia | 60 | 6.2 | $2485 |
| 196 | Columbia | 260 | 4.9 | $1735 |
| 197 | Columbia | 25 | 5.1 | $1505 |
| 198 | Columbia | 150 | 4.4 | $940 |

## 15-7: RETURN ON INVESTMENT

A hospital is considering purchase of a home health agency. It expects to net $175,000 income each year for the next 10 years. The purchase price of the agency is $1.1 million, and the hospital's required rate of return is 7 percent.

### Questions:

1. Is this investment project wise?
2. What is the payback period for the home health agency purchase?
3. What is the average rate of return for the home health agency purchase?

## 15-8: PERSONAL BALANCE SHEET

### Scenario:

Personal financial information as of 3/31/200x:
- Checking account balance $800
- Credit union account balance $1,100
- Department store bill $350
- Credit card bill $555
- All other bills for this month have been paid

### Home:

Purchase price was $85,000 in 1985.
Remaining principal of $45,000 to Cascade Mortgage.
Monthly mortgage payments are $720.

### Automobile:

Purchase price was $5,000 on preowned model Subaru Legacy 1993
Monthly payments $320.
Amount owed $1,500.

### Retirement Fund:

IRA established last month with a $2,000 deposit.

### Directions:

1. Arrange above information into a balance sheet using the sections illustrated in Chapter 15.
2. State any assumptions made in preparation of the personal balance sheet.

# Review Answers

## PRETEST REVIEW ANSWER KEY

### Directions:

1. Correct your Pretest answers with the answers below by placing a slash through the incorrect question number (Example: 8) with a pen or pencil of a contrasting color.
2. Record the correct answer by placing a square around the letter of the correct answer.
3. Record the total correct on the Initial Performance Grid in Section 4 of this review manual.
4. Calculate your performance rate and also record on the grid.
5. Promptly locate the correct answer for each question missed in the chapter of the textbook.
6. Proceed to the chapter review if your performance rate was 80% or higher; otherwise, return to the chapter for further study.

### Answers to Pretest Review:

| 1. | b | 6. | b |
| 2. | a | 7. | a |
| 3. | b | 8. | a |
| 4. | b | 9. | b |
| 5. | a | 10. | a |

## CHAPTER REVIEW ANSWER KEY

### Directions:

1. Correct your answers with the answers below by placing a slash through the incorrect question number (Example: 8) with a pen or pencil of a contrasting color.
2. Record the correct answer by placing a square around the letter of the correct answer.
3. Record the total correct on the Initial Performance Grid in Section 4 of this review manual.
4. Calculate your performance rate and also record on the grid.
5. Promptly locate the correct answer for each question missed in the chapter of the textbook.
6. Proceed to the next chapter assigned in your study.

### Answers to Chapter Review:

1. d
2. b
3. b
4. b
5. d
6. 2.67 years ($3.00 × 1500) del/yr = $4,500; $12,000/$4,500
7. 2.04 - $2,438,776/$1,197,521
8. (2.078)
   ($2,954,609 – 3,015,774)
   ($61,165)/$2,954,609
9. folders
10. rent

# CHAPTER 16

# TECHNOLOGY, APPLICATIONS, AND SECURITY

## Review

### PRETEST REVIEW

**Directions:**

1. *Read each question carefully before selecting an answer.*
2. *Circle the letter of the correct answer.*
3. *Answer all the questions since there is no penalty for this pretest review.*
4. *Check your answers with the answer key located at the end of this chapter.*

1. COBOL is an example of a 4GL.
   a. True
   b. False

2. An interface engine is responsible for supplying ADT data to clinical systems.
   a. True
   b. False

3. Biometrics is a type of firewall.
   a. True
   b. False

4. "Enterprise-wide" refers to a departmental system.
   a. True
   b. False

5. Business Rules is the name of the software package that resides on an application server.
   a. True
   b. False

6. The Internet Network Foundation regulates the operation of the Internet.
   a. True
   b. False

7. The smaller the bandwidth, the more compact and faster the network transmission.
   a. True
   b. False

8. DRG 483 provides more data granularity than ICD9-CM code 428.0.
   a. True
   b. False

9. A primary key is a field that links tables in a database.
   a. True
   b. False

10. Ethernet refers to a type of telemedicine software.
    a. True
    b. False

# CHAPTER REVIEW

## Directions:

*1. Read each question carefully before selecting an answer.*
*2. Circle the letter of the correct answer.*
*3. Answer all the questions since there is no penalty for this pretest review.*
*4. Check your answers with the answer key located at the end of this chapter.*

1. A CGI script is used to run programs on a computer.
   a. True
   b. False

2. TCP/IP is a communication protocol used for transmitting data over the Internet.
   a. True
   b. False

3. A comprehensive health information system is composed of:
   a. business and financial systems
   b. clinical information systems
   c. departmental systems
   d. all of the above

4. Middleware is a type of software used to support clinical systems such as pharmacy.
   a. True
   b. False

5. When data are combined with analysis tools, the result is called a:
   a. clinical information system
   b. database management system
   c. decision-support system
   d. data-mart
   e. all of the above
   f. none of the above

6. All of the following languages are used to display Web documents EXCEPT:
   a. XML
   b. HTML
   c. SGML
   d. HTTP

7. Patient accounting systems usually follow which database model?
   a. relational
   b. hierarchical
   c. network
   d. object-oriented

8. ATM refers to:
   a. electronic mail
   b. database
   c. network transfer
   d. telemedicine

9. Telemedicine applications include the areas of:
   a. home health services
   b. referral communications center
   c. radiology
   d. b and c
   e. a and c
   f. All of above

10. CODEC is the abbreviation for:
    a. Council of Data Enterprise Collection
    b. Coder-Decoder
    c. Consortium of Data Encryption
    d. none of the above

*Additional review questions can be found on the CD-ROM.*

# Assignments

## 16-1: FORECAST DOCUMENT

Develop a forecast document on anticipated changes in how patient information is exchanged among health care organizations in the next 5 years. The forecast should include:

- Background information on current technology used to transmit health care information
- Factors influencing new technology
- Barriers to implementation

## 16-2: IN-SERVICE PROGRAM ON PROTECTING ELECTRONIC INFORMATION

Prepare an annotated outline for an in-service program for the health information management staff to address the organization's technical policies and procedures on data security.

The program should include:

- Definition of key terms
- Types of methods for encryption and how the Internet handles encryption
- Process of developing revised security policies
- References used

## 16-3: DATA REQUIREMENTS FOR DEVELOPING A DATA MART

### Scenario:

The CEO of 300-bed hospital indicates a need for specific analysis of financial data to help senior management with next year's strategic plan. In particular, they need to understand the demographics of their patient base and some idea of reimbursement patterns.

### Directions:

*Prepare 10 to 15 questions for the CEO to determine the data requirements for this project.*

## 16-4: HTML/XML FACT SHEET

Prepare a question and answer (Q&A) fact sheet that poses questions and answers about HTML and XML for distribution at the annual medical staff retreat on health care computing. Include in this information how these languages can be used in a health care organization.

## 16-5: THOUGHT QUESTIONS

1. Explain how an Intranet could be used within a physician group practice. Discuss the potential types of information that can be made available on the Intranet that would benefit the physician group practice.
2. Discuss the issues involved in a cost-benefit analysis of implementing a telemedicine program in a rural community. List the costs and the benefits—both monetary and nonmonetary?
3. Develop some user-defined tags for use in XML that might be relevant to a Web-based clinical information system. Explain why HTML is difficult to use for this application.
4. Explain how administrative barriers can slow progress in the implementation of health information systems. Cite two areas from the emerging technology section of Chapter 16 where barriers are found and present possible solutions.
5. Choose one type of health information system (departmental, enterprise, etc.) and explain how a role-based access control list would be implemented.
6. List three major strides that occurred in the 1990s that moved the health care industry farther along toward achieving health information systems goals and expectations.
7. Summarize the types of firewall solutions available and provide an example of how one is used in a health care environment.
8. Do you think it is possible to capture too much data with a point-of-care system? Why or why not?
9. Describe how Secure Socket Layer (SSL) transmission works for a standard browser.
10. Explain some of the timeliness of data issues involved with operating a data mart.

# Review Answers

## PRETEST REVIEW ANSWER KEY

### Directions:

1. Correct your Pretest answers with the answers below by placing a slash through the incorrect question number (Example: *8*) with a pen or pencil of a contrasting color.
2. Record the correct answer by placing a square around the letter of the correct answer.
3. Record the total correct on the Initial Performance Grid in Section 4 of this review manual.
4. Calculate your performance rate and also record on the grid.
5. Promptly locate the correct answer for each question missed in the chapter of the textbook.
6. Proceed to the chapter review if your performance rate was 80% or higher; otherwise, return to the chapter for further study.

### Answers to Pretest Review:

| | | | | |
|---|---|---|---|---|
| 1. | b | 6. | a |
| 2. | a | 7. | b |
| 3. | b | 8. | b |
| 4. | b | 9. | a |
| 5. | b | 10. | b |

## CHAPTER REVIEW ANSWER KEY

### Directions:

1. Correct your answers with the answers below by placing a slash through the incorrect question number (Example: *8*) with a pen or pencil of a contrasting color.
2. Record the correct answer by placing a square around the letter of the correct answer.
3. Record the total correct on the Initial Performance Grid in Section 4 of this review manual.
4. Calculate your performance rate and also record on the grid.
5. Promptly locate the correct answer for each question missed in the chapter of the textbook.
6. Proceed to the next chapter assigned in your study.

### Answers to Chapter Review:

| | | | | |
|---|---|---|---|---|
| 1. | a | 6. | d |
| 2. | a | 7. | b |
| 3. | d | 8. | c |
| 4. | a | 9. | f |
| 5. | e | 10. | b |

Copyright © 2001 by W.B. Saunders Company. All rights reserved.

# CHAPTER 17

# Electronic Health Records: A Unifying Principle

## Review

### PRETEST REVIEW

### Directions:

1. *Read each question carefully before selecting an answer.*
2. *Circle the letter of the correct answer.*
3. *Answer all the questions since there is no penalty for this pretest review.*
4. *Check your answers with the answer key located at the end of this chapter.*

1. Which of the following is a science that deals with health information, its structure, acquisition, and uses?
    a. health information
    b. telehealth
    c. medical informatics
    d. health informatics

2. Expected electronic health record functions include:
    a. 24 x 7 availability
    b. links to external databases
    c. access to research databases
    d. a and b
    e. a, b, and c

3. Which of the following describes the formulation of the relationship among elements of data and information?
    a. rules
    b. alerts
    c. knowledge
    d. decision support

4. Transcribed radiology reports and digital diagnostic images in radiology databases can be accessed via a web server using Netscape browser.
    a. True
    b. False

5. Internet-derived technologies are used in applications that communicate:
    a. between individuals in separate organizations using the public transport
    b. between individuals and published websites using public transport
    c. in internal and external applications using public transport and institutional intranets
    d. a and b
    e. a, b, and c

6. The electronic health record includes:
   a. software and hardware
   b. technology infrastructure and communications
   c. multimedia
   d. all of the above

7. The American National Standards Institute coordinates the activities of voluntary standards-setting systems and organizations.
   a. True
   b. False

8. The electronic health record brings together diverse information systems to integrate care and service data.
   a. True
   b. False

9. Interface information systems are characterized by:
   a. a common database shared by all departments
   b. a single data dictionary
   c. both a and b
   d. none of the above

10. What does the Electronic Health Record Content and Structure Standard (E 1384) offer EHR developers?
    a. direction on the scope of content
    b. data content, definitions and formats to help in developing EHR data dictionaries
    c. technical security components for EHR system designers
    d. a & b

# CHAPTER REVIEW

## Directions:

1. Read each question carefully before selecting an answer.
2. Circle the letter of the correct answer.
3. Answer all the questions since there is no penalty for this pretest review.
4. Check your answers with the answer key located at the end of this chapter.

1. Which of the following collects clinical data from diverse sources in an integrated manner and reorganizes it for storage?
   a. data dictionary
   b. data repository
   c. database management system
   d. local area network

2. What do clinical alert features used in the HELP system?
   a. outsourced database review procedures to identify "alert" situations
   b. executive decision support systems
   c. clinical guideline reference look-up for physicians
   d. data-driven rules that interact with physicians

3. Paper records, when combined with electronic health records, lack the ability to serve the health care process because:
   a. the over-all health information process is more complex
   b. most providers have adopted technology and demand it for the record
   c. the information must be available in multiple locations simultaneously
   d. operational costs, the demand for efficient delivery of clinical information, continuity, and availability of technology

4. The organizational trend is to combine analysis and systems design methods, database management, and data standards through interfaced information systems.
   a. True
   b. False

5. Standard communication protocols are required of interface information systems.
   a. True
   b. False

6. A principal disadvantage of integrated information systems is that only departmental employees are authorized to change data.
   a. True
   b. False

7. What kind of health information system meets the needs of users external to the individual organization such as payers, researchers, and planners?
   a. community health information system
   b. distributed health information system
   c. executive information system
   d. integrated health information system

8. A combination of which of the following systems comprise the elements of the technology infrastructure?
   a. business and financial systems
   b. clinical information systems
   c. departmental systems
   d. a & c
   e. all of the above

9. Sponsors of electronic health record systems include those who:
    a. authorize and fund the EHR
    b. oversee and use the systems
    c. lead users in analyzing alternative EHR models
    d. perform technical evaluation of systems

10. A "science that deals with health information, its structure, acquisition and uses" is a definition of:
    a. health information
    b. telehealth
    c. medical informatics
    d. health informatics

*Additional review questions can be found on the CD-ROM.*

# Assignments

## 17-1: CURRENT FORCES IN ELECTRONIC HEALTH RECORD SYSTEMS

Prepare a presentation suitable for the medical record committee of a hospital medical staff on the current forces that are driving growth in electronic health records. The presentation should include approximately 10 to 12 visual aids and/or a two- to three-page outline. Include references or websites that can be used by the committee members to obtain more information about the topics.

## 17-2: FORECAST DOCUMENT

Develop a forecast document on anticipated changes in patient record management in the next ten years. The forecast should include:

- Background information on paper patient records
- Value of electronic health records
- Legal and behavioral milestones

## 17-3: IN-SERVICE PROGRAM ON CONFIDENTIALITY OF ELECTRONIC HEALTH RECORDS

Prepare an annotated outline for an in-service program for the health information management department staff to address the new concerns on patient confidentiality now that more and more of the patient record is electronically based.

The program should include:

- Definitions of key terms.
- Roles of various types of health care professionals, including the health information management department staff, in protecting patients' privacy.
- Electronic means of limiting access to portions of patient records.
- Security measures of protecting integrity of data/information.
- Disciplinary measures for violating privacy or breaching security.
- References used.

## 17-4: PLANNING FOR ELECTRONIC HEALTH RECORDS—HIM ROLE

### Scenario:
A 400-bed hospital has announced they will begin a multiyear project to develop electronic health records. The process is being defined and mapped out in an institutional Information Technology Master Plan. As the health information manager, you are participating in this process.

### Directions:
*Discuss the major components that would be addressed in the master plan. Be sure t consider the big picture.*

## 17-5: ELECTRONIC HEALTH RECORD FACT SHEET

Prepare a fact sheet that poses questions and provides answers about electronic health records. The fact sheet will be distributed at a student presentation on impact of new technology at the state Health Information Management Association meeting.

## 17-6: HEALTH INFORMATICS

Prepare a presentation for a group of health information managers on health informatics. Include the definition of the term and the relationship to patient data processing tasks. Feature the role of electronic health records within the health informatics domain.

## 17-7: PERSONAL STRATEGIC PLAN

### Directions:
1. Review the 12 major tasks that are listed in the Chapter 17 discussion on managing the transition from paper-based patient records to an electronic health record system.
2. Select and record on the worksheet six tasks to formulate for a personal strategic plan.
3. Explain your choices.

## 17-8: ELECTRONIC HEALTH RECORDS SCENARIO

Prepare a scenario that depicts a patient arriving in an emergency department of a health care facility that has an electronic health record project under way. The clinical lab, radiology imaging, pharmacy, master patient index, on-line transcription, and discharge database are part of this electronic system.

## 17-9: FLOWCHARTS FOR THE AMBULATORY HEALTH RECORDS CYCLE

Automating ambulatory health records relies on a fundamental patient information cycle that characterizes ambulatory health care delivery. Prepare flowcharts that illustrate that cycle—one for before and one for after electronic health records are implemented.

## 17-10: THOUGHT QUESTIONS

1. Explain how the progress in developing electronic health records described in Chapter 17 contributes to current expectations.
2. Explain how current developments in communications technology and data exchange standards are likely to support individual patients in the health care delivery process.
3. Explain how specific patient data that are entered into a clinical data repository and combined with special analysis software can generate clinical steps in the care process. Provide an example that illustrates this function.
4. What are the issues and barriers that must be addressed in developing electronic health record systems? How can health information managers address them as a profession?
5. Describe the unique contributions made by the HELP system.
6. Characterize the basic limitation of the paper patient record as identified through the Institute of Medicine Study completed in 1991.
7. Discuss the expectations for electronic health records from a clinician's perspective.
8. Why is technical infrastructure necessary for electronic health records to be developed?
9. Explain why health information processing standards are important to the development of electronic health records.
10. Explain how the current concerns about privacy and confidentiality affect the health information management profession.
11. Describe the information expectations of clinicians due to the availability of health information systems.
12. What is bedside documentation? How does it contribute to increased efficiency for nursing personnel and better documentation for patient records?
13. Explain how patient data are used by clinicians in both day-to-day patient management and in planning for future resources.
14. How can electronic health record systems be used to assess and manage special populations of patients? Give an example.
15. Examine the working assumptions at the end of Chapter 17. Recommend additions or modifications.
16. Chapter 17 in the textbook summarizes common purposes of health information systems. Discuss how these purposes help set the direction for information system planners.

# Review Answers

## PRETEST REVIEW ANSWER KEY

### Directions:

1. Correct your Pretest answers with the answers below by placing a slash through the incorrect question number (Example: *8*) with a pen or pencil of a contrasting color.
2. Record the correct answer by placing a square around the letter of the correct answer.
3. Record the total correct on the Initial Performance Grid in Section 4 of this review manual.
4. Calculate your performance rate and also record on the grid.
5. Promptly locate the correct answer for each question missed in the chapter of the textbook.
6. Proceed to the chapter review if your performance rate was 80% or higher; otherwise, return to the chapter for further study.

### Answers to Pretest Review:

| 1. | d | 6. | d |
| 2. | e | 7. | a |
| 3. | c | 8. | a |
| 4. | a | 9. | d |
| 5. | e | 10. | d |

## CHAPTER REVIEW ANSWER KEY

### Directions:

1. Correct your answers with the answers below by placing a slash through the incorrect question number (Example: *8*) with a pen or pencil of a contrasting color.
2. Record the correct answer by placing a square around the letter of the correct answer.
3. Record the total correct on the Initial Performance Grid in Section 4 of this review manual.
4. Calculate your performance rate and also record on the grid.
5. Promptly locate the correct answer for each question missed in the chapter of the textbook.
6. Proceed to the next chapter assigned in your study.

### Answers to Chapter Review:

| 1. | d | 6. | b |
| 2. | d | 7. | a |
| 3. | d | 8. | e |
| 4. | b | 9. | a |
| 5. | b | 10. | d |

# CHAPTER 18

# INFORMATION SYSTEMS LIFE CYCLE

## Review

### PRETEST REVIEW

### Directions:

1. *Read each question carefully before selecting an answer.*
2. *Circle the letter of the correct answer.*
3. *Answer all the questions since there is no penalty for this pretest review.*
4. *Check your answers with the answer key located at the end of this chapter.*

1. A group process used in the analysis and design of an information system is referred to as GDSS.
   a. True
   b. False

2. A central repository identifying all data in a system is a data store.
   a. True
   b. False

3. Maintenance is one of the usual stages of an Information Systems Life Cycle.
   a. True
   b. False

4. Evaluation is one of the usual stages of a Systems Development Life Cycle.
   a. True
   b. False

5. An entity-relationship diagram illustrates the design of an information system database.
   a. True
   b. False

6. CASE can be helpful in operating an information system.
   a. True
   b. False

7. Development costs are to discounted payback period as investments costs in present dollars are to paycheck period.
   a. True
   b. False

8. The first stage in the system design process is the logical systems design.
   a. True
   b. False

9. RFPs are requested of vendors when entertaining the acquisition or expansion of an information system.
   a. True
   b. False

10. RFPs must contain technical, training, and implementation specifications.
    a. True
    b. False

## CHAPTER REVIEW

### Directions:

1. *Read each question carefully before selecting an answer.*
2. *Circle the letter of the correct answer.*
3. *Answer all the questions since there is no penalty for this pretest review.*
4. *Check your answers with the answer key located at the end of this chapter.*

1. Matrix tables and data flow diagrams are tools useful to the analysis phase in the Systems Design Life Cycle.
   a. True
   b. False

2. Variability in Information Systems Life Cycles can result in a phenomenon called discontinuity.
   a. True
   b. False

3. The maturity phase of the General Systems Life Cycle is similar to which phase in the Information Systems Life Cycle?
   a. growth
   b. implementation
   c. operation and maintenance
   d. obsolescence

4. What are data stores and data flows related to?
   a. data dictionaries
   b. data flow diagrams
   c. decision trees
   d. none of the above

5. Referring to the illustration below, in what component of an information system would you find this notation?

| | |
|---|---|
| **Project:** | Record Completion Review System |
| **Label:** | Daily Discharge List |
| **Entry Type:** | Data Flow |
| **Description:** | Daily list of patients discharged from the hospital |
| **Alias:** | None |
| **Composition:** | Daily Discharge List = current date + medrecno + pt name + pt name + pt midinital + pt dob + admit date + dischg date |
| **Locations:** | Context- and first-level explosions; second-level explosion of Process 1, Record Catalog |
| | Data Flow → Daily Discharge List |

6. CASE is useful in the construction of the:
   a. entity-relationship diagram
   b. data flow diagram
   c. data dictionary
   d. all of the above

7. Information about the process of a data element can be found in each of the following except the:
   a. explosion diagram
   b. data flow diagram
   c. data dictionary
   d. entity-relationship diagram

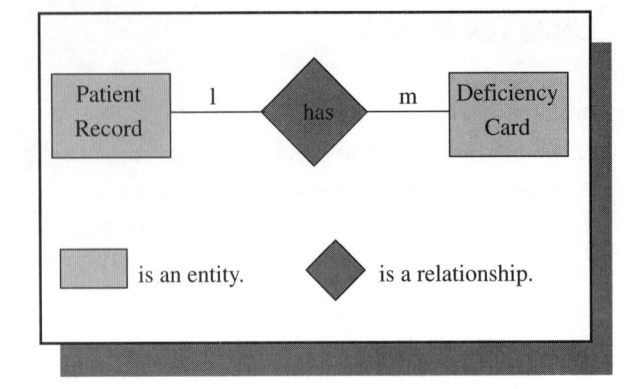

8. Referring to the illustration immediately above, what is the name of this diagram?

9. Referring to the illustration immediately above, "m" means what?

10. Referring to the information in the table below, calculate the cumulative difference in costs. In which year will the payback period be reached?
    a. year 1
    b. year 2
    c. year 3
    d. none of the above

|  | Year 1 | Year 2 | Year 3 |
|---|---|---|---|
| Current System Cost | 16,000 | 16,000 | 16,000 |
| New System Cost | 26,000 | 11,000 | 11,000 |
| Yearly Difference in Costs | -10,000 | +5,000 | +5,000 |
| Cumulative Difference in Costs |  |  |  |

*Additional review questions can be found on the CD-ROM.*

# Assignments

## 18-1: PROFESSIONAL PRACTICE: ANALYSIS OF INFORMATION SYSTEMS LIFE CYCLE STAGE

### Directions:

*In a health information management department, use the attached worksheets to:*

1. Identify all the electronic/computerized systems that are currently used within the department.
2. Identify the electronic/computerized systems that the department interfaces with on an institution-wide level.

### Questions:

1. How do the systems from various facilities compare?
2. Why do the differences exist?
3. Are the Information Systems Life Cycle (ISLC) stages correct? Why or why not?

### Optional Addition to Above Assignment:

Obtain a copy of the HIM Department's strategic plan. Assess whether the departmental information systems support the strategic objectives. Justify your analysis.

## 18-1: WORKSHEET: ANALYSIS OF INFORMATION SYSTEMS LIFE CYCLE

*Complete a separate worksheet for each system.*

| | |
|---|---|
| System name: | |
| Department location: | |
| Age of system: | |
| Functionality – Output and functions: | |
| Hardware platform: | |
| Software platform: | |
| Interfaces with or stand alone: | |
| ISLC stage: | |
| Rationale for selection of ISLC stage: | |

## 18-2: HIERARCHY AND DATA FLOW DIAGRAM

*Construct a hierarchy chart and data flow diagram for the physician chart completion process listed below:*

### Physician Completion Process

1. Physician requests incomplete records.
2. Pull physician deficiency data card from Deficiency Card File.
3. Pull incomplete records from Incomplete Record File Area.
4. Give records to physician.
5. Physician completes records.
6. Physician returns records to HIM staff.
7. HIM staff reviews records to determine if physician completed all deficiencies.
8. HIM staff removes deficiencies noted on physician deficiency data cards.
9. If deficiencies still exist for same physician, HIM staff refiles records in Incomplete Record File Area.
    A. Makes new deficiency card.
    B. Attaches one copy of card to patient's record.
    C. File copy of deficiency card in physician Deficiency Card File.
10. If physician completed all deficiencies, check for additional deficiency cards attached to record. If additional deficiency cards are present, file record in Incomplete Record File Area.
11. If no deficiencies exist, file record in Permanent File.

## 18-3: PROFESSIONAL PRACTICE: HIERARCHY CHART AND DATA FLOW DIAGRAM

### Directions:

1. At a health care facility, investigate an HIM function assigned by the instructor.
2. Document the process in Narrative, Hierarchy Chart and Data Flow Diagram formats. Refer to the Record Completeness Review Example in Chapter 18.

### Questions:

1. What problems did you encounter in developing the structured tools?
2. What benefits were gained by utilizing structured tools?
3. How can you improve proficiency in using these tools?

## 18-4: PROFESSIONAL PRACTICE: DATA DICTIONARY

### Directions:

*Develop a data dictionary for the function and system studied in Assignment 18-3. Include definitions for all data elements, data stores, data flows, and data processes. Use the format as specified in Chapter 18.*

### Questions:

If the same system at different facilities is studied by the group, compare the data dictionaries. Identify the reasons or rationales for the differences.

## 18-5: INTERVIEW PROTOCOL

### Scenario:

One of the strategic objectives of Community Hospital is to improve the quality of patient care. To support this objective, a more comprehensive information system is required. A steering committee has been appointed to lead the process of investigation, analysis, and design of the new system to support continuous quality improvement. A subcommittee has been assigned the task of developing a draft of the interview protocol and identifying the interview audience.

### Directions:

*Develop the following deliverables and present them for review and critique by the subcommittee:*

1. Characteristics of the interview audience.
2. General purpose and goals of the interviews.
3. Interview protocol including structured and unstructured questions.
4. Brief rationale for the inclusion of each question in the protocol.
5. Brief description of how responses to each question will be tabulated and analyzed.
6. Brief description of expected summary results.

## 18-6: QUESTIONNAIRE TO ASSESS INTERFACE FUNCTIONALITY

### Scenario:

Community Hospital plans to replace its current hospital information system. One part of the process is the design of the functional requirements for admitting, emergency services, and clinic interfaces to the master patient index. You are a member of the functional requirements development team and have been assigned the task of determining user satisfaction with the current system and what enhanced features or functionality is desired.

### Directions:

*Develop a survey instrument to assess current interface functionality. The deliverables of this project include:*

1. Description of survey purpose and goals.
2. Identification of target audience.
3. Preparation of cover letter to go with the questionnaire.
4. Development of questions and survey instrument.
5. Discussion of how data will be tabulated and analyzed.

## 18-7: IMPLEMENTATION PLAN

### Scenario:

The health information management department at Community Hospital will be implementing the system studied in Assignments 18-3 and 18-4. This function is not currently computerized in the department.

### Assignment:

Develop an implementation plan for installing this system in the department. The plan should include discussion and specifics about:

- User preparation
- Site preparation
- System testing
- System conversion
- System startup

## 18-8: PHYSICIANS' COLLECTION AGENCY

### Scenario:

The Physicians' Collection Agency is owned and operated cooperatively by several hundred solo and small group medical practices in the Southwest. Each member of the agency pays a fee for each credit report received from Physicians' and a percentage is paid to the agency for each bad debt collected. Costs are maintained at a level sufficiently high to cover the costs of operation. The agency maintains a file of the credit experience of most patients of the physician members and works closely with the retail credit agencies in the areas where it operates. It functions as an intermediary for the business managers of the various practices, who can call the agency on a special telephone line and obtain ratings on credit of present and prospective patients as well as providing collection services.

Physicians' Collection Agency is organized into four departments: reporting, investigation, collection, and administrative services. The reporting department is responsible for reading files over the telephone when merchants call for immediate information upon which to base credit decisions. The investigation department functions primarily to verify credit references given by prospective customers. It also updates credit files that have been inactive for a long period when requests are received for reactivating them.

The collection department, as the name implies, assists members in collecting overdue debts. Finally, administrative services does the printing and other supportive work necessary for the proper functioning of the other departments. It also is responsible for the agency's sales function, which is designed to enlist new members who can utilize the firm's services.

Three years ago Howell Ray, the president of the agency, with the approval of the board of directors, employed a national company to design and install a comprehensive management information system. The primary goal was to improve internal control by supplying information that would assist all departments in more effectively coordinating their operations. The system would also provide Ray with overall operating data used to develop long-range plans and policies. One year after the firm was hired, an operational information system was functioning at Physicians' Collection Agency.

In the two years since the system was installed, the agency's computer has printed thousands of pages of information concerning operations. Some of the reports go to the president and department heads weekly and some monthly, and a few are compiled quarterly. The reports range from estimated operating costs, to days of work lost due to illness, to projected productivity figures. The cost of the computer rental and operation is now one of the agency's major expenditures.

In spite of the new information, President Ray sees little improvement in departmental operations. Everyone seems to function as they did before the information system was installed. Even Ray rarely reads the printouts he receives, although he has his secretary summarize them, circulate the summaries to department heads, and file them for future reference.

Ray decided to find out why no one uses the data supplied by the computer. He circulated a memorandum to department heads asking if the computer services are being used in coordinating departmental operations. If so, what benefits are being received? If not, what are the reasons for the lack of use?

As the responses came in an interesting pattern developed. Without exception, all managers stated that they felt the computer was potentially valuable but not as it was presently being utilized. A few of the more representative comments and reactions are listed below.

- "The type of information I receive is not the type needed to improve operations. No one ever asked me what I really needed."

- "After two years I still cannot understand what the printout says. It is just a lot of numbers so far as I can see."
- "All I do is receive computer reports and no one mentions them. What am I supposed to do once they come to me?"
- "One thing is quite evident, the reports are inaccurate. Periodically, I run trial checks on selected portions of the data, and the printouts simply do not conform to what I know to be actual conditions. I am afraid to use them."

Ray, although disappointed, was not surprised. He felt essentially the same as his department heads. Now he really did not know what to do.

## Questions:

1. From the comments received in response to President Ray's memo, what is your reaction to the Physicians' Collection Agency information system?
2. How do you think a situation such as this could develop?
3. What are Ray's alternative courses of action at this point? What do you think he should do? Why?

# Review Answers

## PRETEST REVIEW ANSWER KEY

### Directions:

1. Correct your Pretest answers with the answers below by placing a slash through the incorrect question number (Example: 8) with a pen or pencil of a contrasting color.
2. Record the correct answer by placing a square around the letter of the correct answer.
3. Record the total correct on the Initial Performance Grid in Section 4 of this review manual.
4. Calculate your performance rate and also record on the grid.
5. Promptly locate the correct answer for each question missed in the chapter of the textbook.
6. Proceed to the chapter review if your performance rate was 80% or higher; otherwise, return to the chapter for further study.

### Answers to Pretest Review:

| | | | | |
|---|---|---|---|---|
| 1. | b | | 6. | b |
| 2. | b | | 7. | b |
| 3. | a | | 8. | a |
| 4. | b | | 9. | b |
| 5. | a | | 10. | a |

## CHAPTER REVIEW ANSWER KEY

### Directions:

1. Correct your answers with the answers below by placing a slash through the incorrect question number (Example: 8) with a pen or pencil of a contrasting color.
2. Record the correct answer by placing a square around the letter of the correct answer.
3. Record the total correct on the Initial Performance Grid in Section 4 of this review manual.
4. Calculate your performance rate and also record on the grid.
5. Promptly locate the correct answer for each question missed in the chapter of the textbook.
6. Proceed to the next chapter assigned in your study.

### Answers to Chapter Review:

| | | | | |
|---|---|---|---|---|
| 1. | a | | 6. | d |
| 2. | a | | 7. | d |
| 3. | c | | 8. | entity-relationship diagram |
| 4. | b | | 9. | many |
| 5. | data dictionary | | 10. | c |

# SECTION III

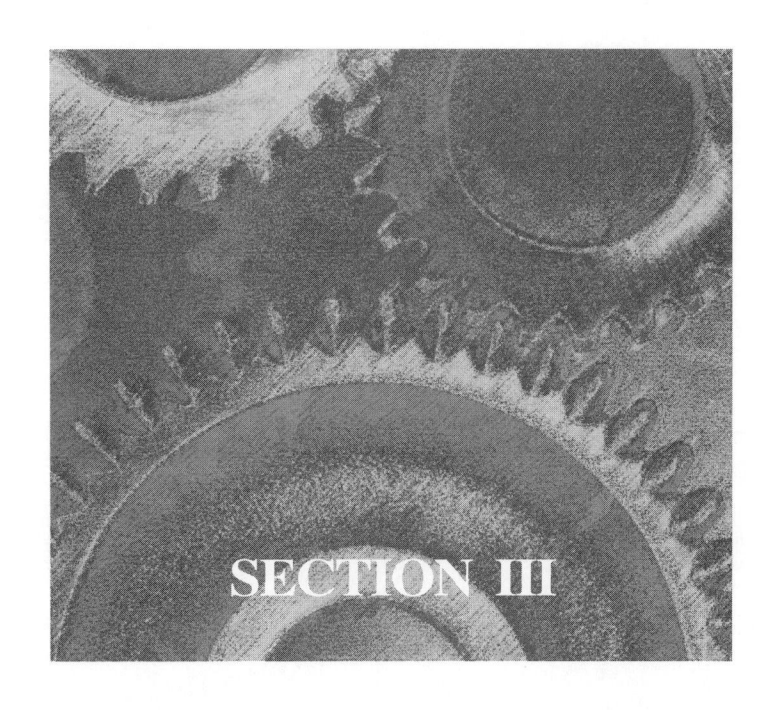

# HOW TO PREPARE FOR CERTIFICATION

# Introduction and Application

Certification is a process of testing a graduate's entry-level knowledge and competence in Health Information Management. The certification examinations for Registered Health Information Technicians (RHIT) and Registered Health Information Administrators (RHIA) are written by the American Health Information Management Association (AHIMA) and are administered by a testing agency once a year in the fall.

Successful passing of the respective examination certifies the graduate for practice at the entry level throughout the United States, Canada, and Puerto Rico. This entrance level is described in the Domains, Tasks, and Subtasks, published by AHIMA and included in Section One of this Study Guide. Successful completion of the respective examination authorizes an individual to use the initials RHIT or RHIA following his or her name. This credential can be retained and used as designated so long as the individual satisfies specified continuing education requirements of AHIMA.

Each certification examination can be taken in any one of 53 testing sites located throughout the United States and Puerto Rico and by special arrangement at other sites in or outside of the United States. These sites may change from year to year.

## Current Testing Center Sites

| State | City | State | City |
|---|---|---|---|
| AK | Anchorage | NC | Charlotte |
| AL | Birmingham | ND | Fargo |
| AR | Little Rock | NE | Omaha |
| AZ | Tempe | NH | Concord |
| CA | Los Angeles | NJ | Clark |
| CA | Oakland | NM | Albuquerque |
| CO | Denver | NY | New York |
| CT | New Haven | NY | Syracuse |
| FL | Jacksonville | OH | Columbus |
| FL | Miami | OK | Oklahoma City |
| FL | Tampa | OR | Portland |
| GA | Atlanta | PA | Philadelphia |
| IA | Iowa City | PA | Pittsburgh |
| ID | Boise | PR | Rio Piedras |
| IL | Chicago | SC | Columbia |
| IN | Indianapolis | SD | Sioux Falls |
| KY | Louisville | TN | Nashville |
| LA | Baton Rouge | TX | Dallas |
| MA | Boston | TX | Houston |
| MD | Baltimore | TX | San Antonio |
| ME | Bangor | UT | Salt Lake City |
| MI | Ann Arbor | VA | Richmond |
| MN | Minneapolis | VT | Burlington |
| MO | Kansas City | WA | Seattle |
| MO | St. Louis | WI | Milwaukee |
| MS | Jackson | WV | Huntington |
| MT | Great Falls | | |

Copyright © 2001 by W.B. Saunders Company. All rights reserved.

Each graduate makes application to write the examination for the field of study in which he or she is a graduate. Application can be made after graduation by writing to the address below. Most college and university programs provide applications for their graduates for first-time testing.

Candidate Services Department
Attention: AHIMA Examinations
8310 Nieman Road
Lenexa, KS 66214
(913) 541-0400
Fax: (913) 541-0156

## Certification Guide Contents

All applicants will receive a Certification Guide for the examination for which they have applied that provides detailed information about the examination:

Calendar of examination activities
General examination information
The application procedure
Examination administration
Examination results and scoring
General information on certification
Examination content
Sample questions

# Certification Examination Content

Each examination consists of multiple-choice questions requiring only one correct answer. Examination questions measure the recall of knowledge, the application of knowledge, and the resolution of problems.

### Knowledge and Comprehension Questions

This involves the recall of a wide range of material from specific facts to complete theories. It may involve translating material from one form to another (words to numbers), by interpreting material, and by predicting consequences or effects.

### Application Questions

This may include the application of such things as rules, methods, concepts, principles, laws, formulas, theories and standards

### Analysis and Problem Solving Questions

This may include the interpretation of information, determining appropriate courses of action, and recognizing relationships.

The examinations are in two parts:

Part I: HIM Competencies
Part II: Coding Competencies

## Certification Examination Cost

The application fee for the examination may change from year to year. A fee of $175.00 for members and $225.00 for nonmembers is currently assessed, payable by check, money order or Visa/MasterCard.

## Certification Examination Scoring

Each examination uses a standard answer sheet like the one shown on the following page. The examinations are machine scored by the testing agency, giving equal weight to all the test questions. Although each examination has two sections, passing or failing is determined from the total number of correct responses on the entire examination.

Examinees receive their test results between 4 and 6 weeks following the examination. Approved applicants may retake the examination, as often as they wish to make application, until they achieve a passing score.

## Preparing for Certification—Before the Exam

1. Begin your review well in advance of the examination. You might review your textbooks and classroom materials first, then practice by re-examining yourself on all chapters (by retaking all Pretests and Chapter Review tests) Or, you may wish to take each review test first, then use your notes and references for further study.

2. Avoid looking at the answers in the Answer Keys while completing each set of review questions.

3. Leave items you cannot answer until you have completed both sets of questions. Then go back and try to answer those left blank. Sometimes other questions will provide clues or information essential for answering a question correctly that you have skipped.

4. Read questions and possible answers carefully. Look for key words, such as "always," "never," "all," "except ," "least," "best," and "not."

5. Do not look for clues to correct answers such as a pattern, or a length of a response, for these are invalid and/or controlled in test construction.

6. Know the location of your scheduled testing site. This information is provided by the testing agency a few weeks before the examination. If possible, it would be wise to make the trip to the site so that you can become familiar with the route and driving conditions (traffic). Locate the exact building, testing room, and bathroom. Pay particular attention to parking locations and parking rules, and to the length of time it took you to drive to the required location.

7. Reread "Test-Taking Principles" in Section One and all of Section Three, "How to Prepare for Certification." The former will refresh your memory about test taking, and the latter will remind you of what you must take to the testing site for admittance.

(The ParSCORE™ form is a product of the Scantron Corporation. ParSCORE is a trademark of Scantron Corporation. Scantron is a registered trademark.)

8. Eat a high-protein, low-fat breakfast before leaving for the testing site. You will not be given a lunch break; the total test time goes through the lunch hour. A high-carbohydrate breakfast generally makes you hungry early (possibly hypoglycemic); a high-fat breakfast may make you drowsy.

## Preparing for Certification—During the Exam

1. Do not burden yourself by taking textbooks and papers into the testing site because they are not allowed in the examination room, except for coding textbooks.

2. Listen carefully to the examination directions given by the test proctor; read carefully the written instructions on the test book when distributed. Be sure of when you are allowed to proceed to Part II of the examination.

3. Skip and mark questions in both the test booklet and on the answer sheet that you want to return to. If time permits, return to those questions. It is better to guess than to leave an item blank.

4. Do not be distracted by how fast others around you may be performing. Concentrate on your own performance and use of time.

5. Review your work on the answer sheet carefully before submitting to the test proctor. Are all

## SECTION IV

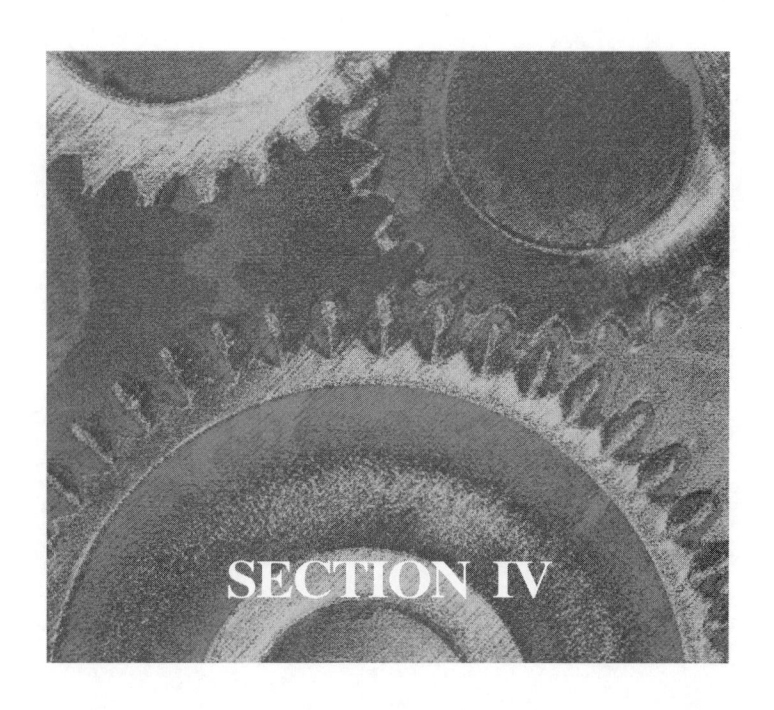

# HOW TO INTERPRET YOUR EXAMINATION READINESS

# Using Performance Grids

This section includes three performance grids:
- The Initial Performance Grid to use upon chapter-by-chapter completion of the Study Guide.
- Repeat Performance Grids for subsequent reviews, perhaps, a final examination, or for certification examination review after graduation.
- Overall Performance Grid. Once you have completed this Study Guide and have filled in data on your performance grid, you can graph your performance for a visual display of your overall competence assessment. Upon doing this, notice in the example below, your performance can be displayed against a "standard" or "goal" which you can determine for yourself:

## Overall Performance Graph

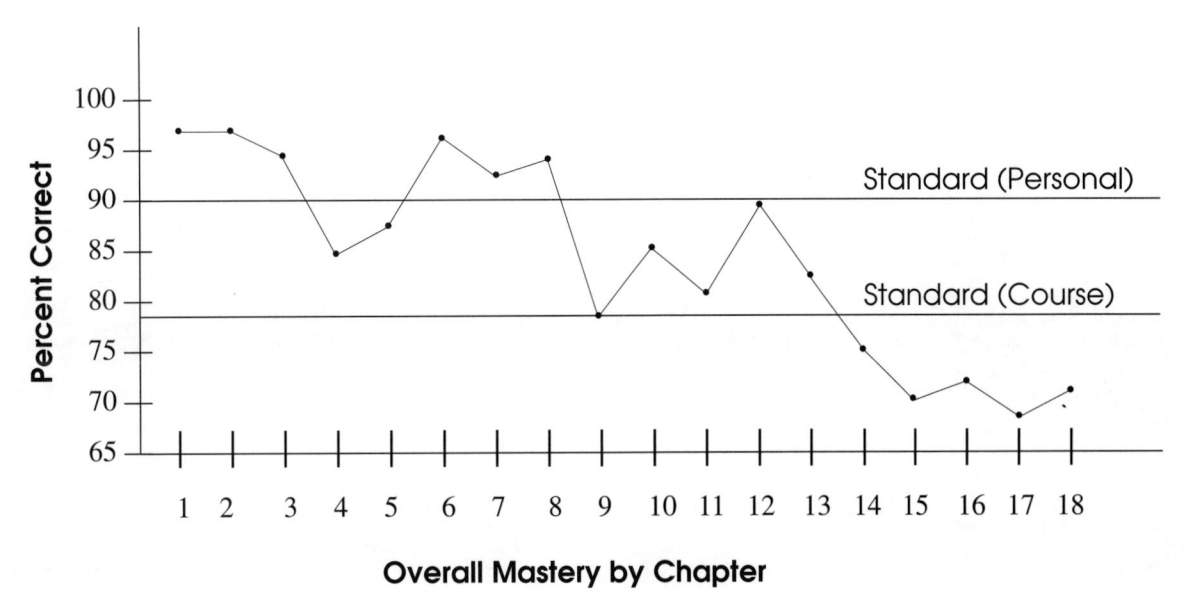

**Overall Mastery by Chapter**

In the above example, a male student set a personal goal of 90% to aim at in striving for mastery of the content. In addition to setting a personal standard, the student drew a horizontal line at 78% denoting what the course standard was for "passing" performance.

Then the student transferred each of the overall mastery percentages from Column 7 in the performance grid to the graph and connected them with straight lines.

Upon self-assessment of his performance against the standards, the student saw that he was successful in achieving "passing" performance in his review work on all the chapters except the last five. He attributed his performance on some of the first chapters in the textbook to their less complex content and decided that, other than a quick overview of that material, no extra effort or time was needed there.

The student considered, but eliminated, the notion that outside classroom activities could not be attributed to his low performance on Chapters 14–18. He attributed his performance solely to the level of difficulty of the material and to the more complex theory that went with the subject matter of the chapters. He decided he needed to do additional exercises in those subjects and to reread the chapters more than once, plus complete some outside recommended reading. He planned to retake the Chapter

Reviews after rereading the chapters and his notes until he achieved his personal goal of 90% on each one. While doing this, he was going to concentrate harder in understanding the underlying principles and reasons for the answers. He planned to use his initial performance graph to display his performance, except that he planned to do it in different colors of ink so that he could more easily analyze his repeated performance against his initial performance.

This student also reminded himself of the context the review questions played in his preparation. He remembered that the questions are few and merely a sampling of the total content. He decided, correctly, that the information in the graph was simply one index of his growing mastery and that he should not be solely dependent on its ability to translate into actual performance on the examination. He decided to add Chapters 9, 10, 11, and 13 to his review study program.

## Initial Performance Grid

| | 1 | 2 | 3 | 4 | 5 | 6 | 7 |
|---|---|---|---|---|---|---|---|
| Chapter | No. of Pretest Questions | No. of Pretest Questions Correct | Percent of Pretest Questions Correct | No. of Chapter Questions | No. of Chapter Questions Correct | Percent of Chapter Questions Correct | Percent Overall Mastery (col2 + col5) 20 |
| 1 | 10 | | | 10 | | | |
| 2 | 10 | | | 10 | | | |
| 3 | 10 | | | 10 | | | |
| 4 | 10 | | | 10 | | | |
| 5 | 10 | | | 10 | | | |
| 6 | 10 | | | 10 | | | |
| 7 | 10 | | | 10 | | | |
| 8 | 10 | | | 10 | | | |
| 9 | 10 | | | 10 | | | |
| 10 | 10 | | | 10 | | | |
| 11 | 10 | | | 10 | | | |
| 12 | 10 | | | 10 | | | |
| 13 | 10 | | | 10 | | | |
| 14 | 10 | | | 10 | | | |
| 15 | 10 | | | 10 | | | |
| 16 | 10 | | | 10 | | | |
| 17 | 10 | | | 10 | | | |
| 18 | 10 | | | 10 | | | |
| Total | 180 | | | 180 | | | |

## Repeat Performance Grid

| Chapter | 1<br>No. of Pretest Questions | 2<br>No. of Pretest Questions Correct | 3<br>Percent of Pretest Questions Correct | 4<br>No. of Chapter Questions | 5<br>No. of Chapter Questions Correct | 6<br>Percent of Chapter Questions Correct | 7<br>Percent Overall Mastery (col2 + col 5) / 20 |
|---|---|---|---|---|---|---|---|
| 1 | 10 | | | 10 | | | |
| 2 | 10 | | | 10 | | | |
| 3 | 10 | | | 10 | | | |
| 4 | 10 | | | 10 | | | |
| 5 | 10 | | | 10 | | | |
| 6 | 10 | | | 10 | | | |
| 7 | 10 | | | 10 | | | |
| 8 | 10 | | | 10 | | | |
| 9 | 10 | | | 10 | | | |
| 10 | 10 | | | 10 | | | |
| 11 | 10 | | | 10 | | | |
| 12 | 10 | | | 10 | | | |
| 13 | 10 | | | 10 | | | |
| 14 | 10 | | | 10 | | | |
| 15 | 10 | | | 10 | | | |
| 16 | 10 | | | 10 | | | |
| 17 | 10 | | | 10 | | | |
| 18 | 10 | | | 10 | | | |
| Total | 180 | | | 180 | | | |

## Overall Performance Grid

| | 1 | 2 | 3 | 4 | 5 | 6 | 7 |
|---|---|---|---|---|---|---|---|
| Chapter | No. of Pretest Questions | No. of Pretest Questions Correct | Percent of Pretest Questions Correct | No. of Chapter Questions | No. of Chapter Questions Correct | Percent of Chapter Questions Correct | Percent Overall Mastery (col2 + col 5) / 20 |
| 1 | 10 | | | 10 | | | |
| 2 | 10 | | | 10 | | | |
| 3 | 10 | | | 10 | | | |
| 4 | 10 | | | 10 | | | |
| 5 | 10 | | | 10 | | | |
| 6 | 10 | | | 10 | | | |
| 7 | 10 | | | 10 | | | |
| 8 | 10 | | | 10 | | | |
| 9 | 10 | | | 10 | | | |
| 10 | 10 | | | 10 | | | |
| 11 | 10 | | | 10 | | | |
| 12 | 10 | | | 10 | | | |
| 13 | 10 | | | 10 | | | |
| 14 | 10 | | | 10 | | | |
| 15 | 10 | | | 10 | | | |
| 16 | 10 | | | 10 | | | |
| 17 | 10 | | | 10 | | | |
| 18 | 10 | | | 10 | | | |
| Total | 180 | | | 180 | | | |